Undelivered

Fertility, Miscarriage And My Journey to Self Compassion

Laura Doyle

Copyright © 2025 by Laura Doyle.

All rights reserved. No part of this book may be used or reproduced in any form whatsoever without written permission except in the case of brief quotations in critical articles or reviews.

This book is not a substitute for professional medical advice, diagnosis, or treatment. The experiences, opinions, and insights shared herein should not be interpreted as medical guidance or as a comprehensive account of all aspects of pregnancy, miscarriage, loss and grief. Readers are advised to consult a qualified medical/healthcare professional or specialist before making any changes to their health care, diet, lifestyle, medication, or treatment plans. Neither the author nor the publisher assumes any liability or responsibility for any loss, injury, or damage incurred as a result of the use or misuse of the information contained in this book.

All names, identifying details, and presentation of individuals and agencies have been changed or anonymised where appropriate to protect privacy. Any resemblance to actual persons, living or dead, is purely coincidental.

ISBN: 978-1-9191909-1-4   Printed in the European Union.

*Book Hub Publishing uses paper sourced only from sustainable forestry. Viva la forests!

We are committed to diversity, inclusion and equality.

Cover design and text layout by Niall MacGiolla Bhuí, ShadowScript Wordsmiths.

CONTENTS

CONTENTS	iii
Prologue	1
Spilling Our Chances	5
Chapter One	6
Chapter Two	12
Chapter Three	13
Chapter Four	20
Chapter Five	23
Chapter Six	36
Chapter Seven	47
Chapter Eight	53
Chapter Nine	63
Chapter Ten	65
Chapter Eleven	68
ChapterTwelve	73
Chapter Thirteen	84
Chapter Fourteen	97
Chapter Fifteen	111
Chapter Sixteen	128
Chapter Seventeen	139
Reflection	148
Dear Me	152
About the Author	157

Acknowledgments 158

Dedication 160

Prologue

This book is for anyone who has had an experience(s) or knows someone who has endured the life-changing grief of infertility, miscarriage, or stillbirth. This includes the anxiety that surrounds people in pregnancy loss or those who have not been graced with the opportunity to experience pregnancy, should they desire it.

Sadly, we all know or will know someone affected by one or all of these issues. With numerous possibilities surrounding the topic of pregnancy, this is not intended to exclude anyone who has experienced trauma in a different way. This is *my* story; therefore, I will speak about what I know. Perhaps it will inspire someone with different experiences to write about them.

I have met and known people who have had losses, but I never understood the significance of fertility issues or miscarriage until I experienced it for myself. I had no insight because nobody readily shares their stories with the public. I respect their choices, but I can no longer stay quiet.

There is a silent epidemic that our society seems to skim over, rarely talking about it, simply because *it's not the done thing* within the constructs of our social order here in Ireland⋯because *it is* an awkward conversation. Meanwhile, women and their significant others are often left to process their losses alone, feeling isolated and forgotten.

I've decided to share my own journey, simply to get important conversations going. My wish is to inform people and introduce new perspectives in the hope that people can feel supported, rather than ignored, during or following this major, life-changing event.

Some people that I know are going to read this and think I'm oversharing. I know this from attempts in the past to open up to friends and family who didn't want to engage. What they don't realise is that I know for a fact that there are people who will definitely get something from this book. Each person's experiences are different, as unique as the way they process any trauma in life. If this book isn't for you, don't read it. It is very detailed in parts and very frank. Anyone who knows me knows that I don't hold back and that I am a straight talker. If you are easily offended or think this is a topic that should not be discussed, move on. For those of us who want to discuss, share, comfort, and inform one another, the time is now.

My husband, Mel, and I have spoken countless times about my initial reservations about speaking up and speaking out. I have confided in him my fears, how I am anxious about saying what I want to say without hurting people, leaving people out, or being considered a bitch. The reality, however, is that we live in a world, where no matter what the intention, someone is probably going to get upset or offended.

This is an account of my experience through my perspective; therefore, if exposing a reality that does not appear true for you, the reader, so be it. Others observing what I went through saw our journey through a completely different lens than us, but the person who was there, who lived through this with me, remains my number one supporter: Mel. For him, for this painfully ugly chapter in the story of us, this personal account of our darkest moments, deserves to be shared.

The idea of having a baby was never at the top of the list for either of us. We partied hard, had lots of holidays, nights away, and always put ourselves first in that regard. But something happened. As I got older, the 'so-called' biological clock started to tick and, my goodness, the tick became a resounding boom in the end.

Mel and I are very fortunate and were in a good position financially and career-wise when we built our modest home between 2019 and 2020. Thankfully, we had just moved into the new house in February of 2020, just one month before the Covid lockdowns and the massive price hikes in the housing market that went along with it.

When the hysteria began to settle, we got married after nearly twenty amazing, fun, and loving years of courtship. We have always been very close, spending all of our free time in each other's company. To this day, it's the same as it was at the start as far as the love is concerned. However, the footprints of grief on our hearts from the challenges of the last few years will always remain.

As with life and every relationship, there are highs and lows. No more than anyone else, we have submerged into the depths, barely able to keep our heads above the despair, but somehow, we always seem to make it through. Life, as they say, is a rollercoaster, and this story is a very detailed, honest, open, and vulnerable account that offers an in-depth look at the reality of our bumpy journey of trying to start a family, mixed in with all of the other challenges that life throws at you in general. For something that is meant to be so 'natural,' attempting to get pregnant really tested us. We were forced to take a serious look at our own mental health, the emotions of grief, sorrow and loss; lack of support and acknowledgement from those close to us. Disappointments and failures of the health care system in Ireland, both public and private, fertility testing, and terminology, procedures, bodily functions, bodily fluids of all sorts, feelings of isolation and thinking that we were losing our minds.

Mel and I have faced the physical and mental consequences of this journey, but we can't be the only ones who struggled. In fact, I know we're not. From speaking to people, I have truly established that this topic is not always treated with the sympathy, understanding, compassion, and recognition that it deserves. For a subject of such a sensitive nature, it is most often brushed under the carpet.

Spilling Our Chances

I washed my hands and sat down at the dressing table. I got the first needle head, and I drew back the fluid and added it to the dissolvable powder. I changed the needle to the finer one and drew up the solution, ready to go. I held it up to tap out any air bubbles, and the liquid was far up the syringe, so I decided to **pull back the plunger a little more.**

The next thing I knew, the part you drew back was in my hand, and the syringe was on the floor. The precious hormone liquid was on me and now on the floor. I froze for a minute, followed by a yell from the bottom of my lungs, screaming, "Noooooooo, no, no, no, no, no." Mel came running down; he had no idea what had happened. I was on my knees on the ground crying and saying, "I spilled it, I spilled it, Mel…I have ruined our chances again."

I wasn't thinking straight. I panicked and I was trying my best to draw it up off the floor into the needle again in sheer desperation. We only had two more attempts after this month with the prescription we had, and I literally just spilled our hopes for that month on the floor…

Chapter One

In my opinion, treatment and care around the entire fertility/pregnancy journey *are not good enough;* it is as simple as that. I know that there are people out there who are currently addicted to peeing on sticks, checking cervical mucus charts and stretchiness, and monitoring if the opening of their cervix is open (well done if you can find it, because I never could). There are women constantly checking apps for ovulation predictions, waiting for the smiley face on those tests to know it's all systems go for the next few days. There are couples obsessed with estimating the possible date when a pregnancy test will potentially read positive, marked with those two lines or that big plus symbol of victory.

Many spend time reading about evaporation lines and false positives, holding tests as close as possible to a light to see if there is even a glimmer of hope. Not to mention assessing temperatures every morning from the bed before moving a muscle in order to look for that slight change in temperature to indicate approaching ovulation.

There are women who wake up in tears at the arrival of 'Aunt Flo,' yet again, and still have to show up for work, knowing that the struggles will continue for at least another month. And there are women who face the day knowing they are losing, or have just lost, a baby—waiting on test results to confirm the worst, bleeding in silence as they carry on. There are women having to inject themselves with hormones, many women are riddled with stress and anxiety, researching the optimal position during sex to make sure that they have the best chance possible, searching online for suggestions such as, "Does lying with your legs above your head after unprotected sex help you to get pregnant?" There are women feeling desperation, alienation, and resentment, coupled with a heavy dose of guilt, when one of those soul-crushing, God-forsaken baby announcements comes through the door or pops up on social media. And once again, it's just not something that you can safely talk about, yet it is so profound amongst women today. It becomes all-consuming when you are in the thick of it. I know, because I was that woman. For the record, I am not saying that the way I have done things is the 'right' way, or that anyone reading this should do it any particular way because I said so. I do not have a medical background nor a degree in any of the specialist areas mentioned in this book; however, all I can do is share what I have learned, what I have done, and what did and didn't work for us. Ultimately, how we dealt with things. I really want to highlight that this is not written as a pity story, rather as a real insight into a tangible experience that I know many other women share with me. Consider this reassurance that you are not alone. I often felt that I had nobody to turn to aside from Mel, as if I wasn't allowed to talk about these things in case I made someone else feel uncomfortable. I felt that nobody really understood what I was talking about and that I was left to plod along when people didn't want to engage in the conversation.

My friends hadn't experienced the things I was going through, as far as I was aware, so I felt (rightly or wrongly) that I couldn't offload because of a perceived lack of understanding or relatability.

My family didn't really address the elephant in the room, not because they didn't want to or were being deliberately avoidant, but probably because they simply didn't know how to approach Mel and me. Some family members did check in with me, and did offer a space to talk and reach out, but I needed more, and even I didn't realise it. I needed someone to reach in and take me by the hand and give me a hug, listen to my woes, hand me the tissues to soak up my tears, and wipe the endless snot away. I needed someone to give me some sympathy if I am being honest. Someone to tell me, "That's really shit and I am so sorry that this happened to you," and to come to be by my side willingly and without having to be invited or asked. Someone to be present for me, acknowledge me and my feelings, and reassure me that I am allowed to talk about it as many times as I needed to without feeling like a plague or a burden. Someone who would allow me to feel how I felt, out loud and in the open. In fact, it's probably my own fault to some degree; I probably kept it all under wraps for quite some time until it finally came pouring out, and they probably didn't realise the heartache that Mel and I were going through.

I was always confident, motivated and determined – if there is something I want, I usually make sure it happens. This is the one thing that I could not control, and it knocked the socks off me. As always, I felt that I had to be the independent, capable, and strong person that I have always been and sort it out for myself in my own way, when all I really needed was to be offered basic support and nurturing without having to seek it out. Overall, that didn't really happen for me, not the way that I needed anyway. I have never been as vulnerable and never felt so alone.

I wish I had somewhere to turn to, to know I wasn't alone. Fertility issues and pregnancy loss are all very common in Ireland today and across the world, but I feel that all-too-few people have those conversations. It's like you are meant to just forget about all of the hurt and sadness, stress and struggles, and just move on because everyone has their own stuff going on. I know from speaking to other people who have experienced or are currently experiencing difficulties in this way that there are common themes that keep recurring, which were also part of my experience. This makes me think that so many women feel the same or similar and *that's why we need to talk.*

I never truly experienced mental health issues until this time in my life, and I tried so hard to get help. I simply couldn't find it for a while, and during those dark days waiting for someone to acknowledge and help me, I had my first and only encounter with suicidal thoughts. I never want to experience that again, nor should anyone experience it due to a lack of help and support. This made me think about all of the people out there who are struggling, wishing and hoping, all of the people who have tried so hard and lost their spark because of negative tests, perceived poor treatment, and lack of full guidance in medical establishments, both public and private.

I also feel that I need to state with profound respect and consideration that my experience is so very, very mild compared to many other women trying to start a family or fulfil their dreams of having children. If that is you and you are reading this, I realise that there are no words that can heal your hurt, anxiety, and sense of loss. You may read this and think, "What the hell is she complaining about? She didn't have to have all of the treatments I've had, or she didn't lose as many tiny heartbeats as I did. She didn't lose a baby at full term or lose precious and costly embryos." So please don't read this thinking I believe I'm the most hard-done-by person out there, because I know I'm not. I'll never truly understand what some people are going through, experiencing, or living, nor will I try to pretend I do. This book is just a conversation starter to try to help people to understand it more and to encourage people to talk about it. So many women experience this kind of loss, turmoil, or face fertility issues to varying degrees. This is my experience, my feelings, and my thoughts.

Our partners play a major role in all of this too, regardless of whether they are a man or a woman, gay or straight. Very often, the husbands and partners are left to wing it. Much depends on the kind of person you're with: are they as invested in this as you are? Is this really what you both want? Is the partner supportive and caring, or do they not seem to care that much? Let's not forget that the partner is needed, after all, to plant the seed, so to speak (not in all cases, mind you). At the time, I worried Mel might get sick of me, because I was basically becoming a sad, anxious, and depressed woman. Thankfully, he stuck with me, and more than that, he lived through it alongside me. Too often, I feel, the partner's feelings and experiences are overlooked.

People often don't realise the mental load carried by those trying to get pregnant or the physical demands in some cases. I've learned a lot, including the importance of keeping your wits about you when facing some of these apparently disinterested consultants in whom you're placing your trust. You need to be well-informed, able to spot any inconsistencies, or recognise their lack of real investment in you and your family. You need to be able to call them out, but also recognise that knowledge is power in the context of advocating for yourself, and that all health and medical personnel have invested a significant amount of time and finance in their education and training. Nonetheless, the more you stand your ground, the better the treatment will be for everyone.

This journey stripped away many of my strong(er) personality traits and characteristics. I became anxiety-ridden, worried excessively about what others would think, and I had low self-esteem. For the first time in my life, I felt like a failure. I was so unhappy, tired, worn out, vulnerable, naïve, and lost. I felt unheard, depressed, and even questioned my sanity. I felt guilty over taking the morning-after pill when I was young and foolish. I questioned what I did to deserve this pain I was feeling and wondered if I was a bad person. I was crying constantly and isolating myself. I spent hours and hours daily searching online, trying to find a solution to fix the 'problem' as I then saw it. I stopped exercising and lost my appetite for both food and life.

So, here is our story, just one of many stories of those living through their own difficulties. Let's talk, people! Whether you are the person trying for a baby, the partner or husband, the family member or friend unsure of what to say or do to help, or someone who simply wants to educate yourself in case you encounter a colleague or loved one going through something similar, arm yourself with some empathy through knowledge.

Chapter Two

Why am I writing this book?

Sadly, we all know or will know someone affected by some of these things. The March of Dimes, an organisation that works on maternal and child health, indicates a miscarriage rate of 10-15% in women who knew they were pregnant. This is not just a problem in Ireland, but a global issue that is not spoken about or supported enough. It's not being given its place, despite the emotional, physical, and mental destruction that it can cause. The WHO comments that miscarriages and stillbirths are not systemically recorded, even in developed countries, suggesting that the numbers could be even higher.

So, why are we not talking about it? The experiences we go through and the emotions we feel may differ for each person, but the wish and the dream are for the same outcome!

Chapter Three

Back in 2013, I was between my Bachelor of Arts degree and my Master's degree (as a mature student) and worked in a local supermarket. I was scanning items through the till for a customer. He was an older man who decided to ask me a series of questions about where I was from and who my relations were. He asked me, "Do you have any children?" and I thought to myself for a moment and chose to reply saying, "I couldn't be telling you everything about me now without asking you a bit about yourself" and I smiled at him. He then said, "Oh, never mind so" and went on about his day. Each week when he came back for his shopping, he came back to me at the till and asked more and more questions about my neighbours and all sorts of other life related questions. I remember telling Mel, my fiancé at the time, that this man was really annoying, as he was asking far too much about me, and I remember saying, "If he keeps asking me if I have children, I'm going to leave him speechless so he will stop asking me."

Lo and behold, a week passed, and there he was again. I was very quiet and didn't really answer his questions until he asked me, "So, are you ever going to tell me if you have a family of your own?" I stopped, looked at him and replied, "You really shouldn't be asking a stranger those sorts of questions, for all you know, I might not be able to have children, did you ever think about that?" Needless to say, there was a short silence, and he answered, "Alright, ok, well you didn't have to be rude like that," and he left the shop. Funny, he didn't come to me at the tills anymore after that. Little did I know what was in store for us when the time came that we would start trying for a baby.

Mel and I have been together for over 23 years. We got together in the summer of 2002 at a house party. I'll give you a flavour of that first night to give you an insight into us as a couple. Our friends' parents had gone away for the night and taken the smaller kids with them, so he threw a party. It was mighty fun. Mel pushed me around on a toy tractor with a trailerload of cans around the house so I could deliver drinks to everyone. I remember being sober the next morning, and it was a lot harder to make conversation than the night before. So, I offered to make tea. I really wanted to get it right. I handed out the tea to everyone and sat down. Some time passed, and I said to Mel, "I didn't see you drinking your tea," and he replied that it was lovely and that he had it all gone. A number of months later, I discovered that he hated it and poured it into the plant pot at the end of the couch. He didn't want to hurt my feelings so he didn't say anything. He was a nice guy from the start.

Jumping forward, we were due to get married in 2020, but due to Covid, this was postponed. Over the years, we had several conversations about starting a family and how many kids we might like. We even discussed what we would do in certain scenarios and laughed over who would be the 'good cop' and the 'bad cop'. Mel, of course, said he would be the strict one. I always laughed when he said that because he is just too nice to be the mean one. As for me, some may say it would come naturally for me to be the mean one.

It was only as the original wedding date came and passed that a strong urge to have a baby suddenly presented itself, but we decided to wait until we were married. I was in my mid-thirties, and Mel had just turned forty, so we were no spring chickens. The biological clock began to tick, and I could really feel the urge and desire building out of the blue once that original wedding date came and passed. We still decided to wait until we were married, despite many conversations where we mentioned our worry about our ages and potentially running out of time.

The week before the wedding took place in October 2021, we had the conversation again and decided that this was it. We were ready to give it a shot (quite literally). It almost felt secretive and fun; after so many years, we could just not worry about getting pregnant anymore. If it happened, it happened. Let's just say we had a lot of fun consecrating the marriage!

We were privileged enough to get married in the fabulous Kilronan Castle, a day and a venue that a girl could only dream of. A day we worked very hard for and a day we will always cherish. Years before this, we went for a drive one Sunday and came across Kilronan Castle which was hosting a wedding fair. I sat in the foyer and watched the pretend bride and groom walk around the hotel as they displayed what would happen on the day of a wedding. They were accompanied by a bagpipe player, and I remember sitting there with tears filling my eyes and saying to Mel, "This is it...this is the place...Could you imagine getting married here?" We said that we would love to get married there, but also realised that there would be very little hope, as it was probably very expensive.

I asked for a wedding brochure anyway, out of curiosity. So, for us, this was a really big achievement.

Can I just add that the day of our wedding happened to be the very first day that the Covid restrictions were fully lifted and everyone was in great form, ready for a proper party! The late bar was back in action until 4 am. As one guest said, "It was like bringing calves to pasture for the first time." The whiskey nearly ran dry. Everyone was delighted to be out and seeing friends and family again. On the day of the wedding, I was asked several times, "Oh, will ye start trying for a baby now straight away?" I just laughed and said, "Oh yeah, let's just see."

October, November, and December passed, and still nothing. It was at this stage that I began to wonder what we were doing wrong, because we really were trying hard, so to speak. Dr. Google stepped in, and I searched and searched. I read all about women's cycles and discovered a lot about ovulation and the very few optimal days that you can actually get pregnant in any given month. I guess I was busy being a pain in the arse to my teachers in school and wasn't listening that day, along with many other days! This made me more mindful of my period and cycle length. Each month, I pulled out the calendar on my phone and marked in my period start date and end date. Then the fun began of trying to predict ovulation from there, because, of course, I had only just learned about the very few optimal days to do the act that might lead to pregnancy. That is how limited my knowledge was.

January 2022 came about, and at that time, I remember saying to myself, "Ok, new year, a fresh start, let's get this right and make it happen." I downloaded a period and ovulation tracker app and put in my details. I was able to tell the app that my cycle was 28 days and that my period only lasted 3 or 4 days. It then gave me my next predicted ovulation date. I thought this was great, sure it took the guesswork out of it all. I only really opened the app the first day of my period to put in the start date, which would then tell me a predicted date for ovulation. I kept that date in the back of my mind going forward and made sure to 'do the job' in around that date and the following days.

I started to think about clean eating, cutting out alcohol, and taking supplements. I had been taking fish oils and a prenatal with folic acid in it for months before this. I followed more women's health pages on Instagram than I like to admit. They all had so much information, it's a minefield. I found a nutritionist called 'AOK Nutrition' who is also a herbalist and takes a great interest in women's health. I spent half a day going through her posts and reels, and again, I learned so much. I was going to get a probiotic and all sorts of natural supplements and remedies from her to help balance my hormones and give me some zen. I had a new sense of positivity that this was going to work!!!! I was going to buy some ovulation predictor tests, and then I would be fully in control and know when to get down to business.

I walked into the pharmacy and went to the aisle where they were. I was keeping an eye out to see if anyone was watching me, but I hadn't a clue what I was buying, so I needed to be there for a while to read the boxes. I bought a packet; they were expensive and I couldn't wait to get home and to read the leaflet. All I took from it was that I pee on the test, I wait and hope to see a smiley face (indicating ovulation is approaching) and a flashing smiley face (it's time to party). It took days to get the smiley face. I couldn't understand because the app said I was going to ovulate, but the test indicated that I wasn't ovulating at that time. So, in fact, I became more confused. This was to become an unwelcome pattern.

This led to more frustration. I needed some other way to be sure I was ovulating because I wasn't getting the result I wanted, but still, my period was regular.

February 2022 came, and I thought to myself, ok, ovulation is due around Valentine's Day (according to the app, which I was beginning to check a little more frequently), let's make this a good one. A few weeks passed, and I woke up to my period. This is the first time I was actually a little annoyed that it had come, and I was in a mood for the day. I remember telling Mel I got my period, and he was ok with that. I wasn't ok with it, but I didn't say too much, as I was hoping I wouldn't get it that month.

That evening when we got home from work, we sat down to talk. I needed a cuddle and a chat. I remember asking him, "Are you not disappointed that it still hadn't happened?" and he replied, saying, 'No, I'm not worried at all. Sure, we aren't trying that long, and if it's meant to be, it will be." Where do you think my hormone-driven mind went at that point...of course, questioning, does he even want a baby, is that why it hasn't happened? I asked him, "Do you not really want this? Now is your time to say before it's too late." His response was very loving, but I saw red. He replied, basically telling me that he is very happy with us, our marriage, and relationship, and if a baby comes along, it comes along, and if it doesn't, it doesn't, and that he will still be happy just with us. Rather than hearing him say that he loved me and what we had, all I took from that was that he wasn't fussed about having a baby. Why does the mind twist things on us?

Anyway, February passed and still nothing. That was it. I was going to the doctor to see if there was anything wrong. She did a full NCT and hormone bloods. Thankfully, all of that came back clear, but in the meantime, I came across a post on AOK Nutritions Instagram account that stated that the way they do that blood test isn't accurate because not everyone ovulates on the same days; therefore, it's inaccurate to carry out the test on day 21 for everyone. Some cycles are longer and some cycles are shorter, so this day 21 test wouldn't be accurate unless you have a perfect 28-day cycle. More on this later on.

Oh great, I thought to myself. Now the doctor doesn't even know what she is doing. I questioned her on this because not everyone has the ideal 28-day cycle that all of the tests are based on, and she didn't really want to engage in that conversation, but I kept digging. I asked if it is accurate because not everyone ovulates on day 21; therefore, the tests can miss the changes to the blood. Eventually, she lowered her head towards her chest and said, "Yes, this test is technically flawed, but it is accurate for the majority." She then added that I was fit and healthy and had nothing to worry about. She told me to be patient and, "DONT STRESS." Don't stress, oh yeah, sure thing, I thought to myself. If only it were that easy. Cheers love!

Chapter Four

The struggle with that damned smiley face on the ovulation tests continued. I searched for other ways to find out if you are ovulating or not and discovered… mucus charts.

Ok, ok…so…mucus! This entailed checking what kind of fluid there was at any time. There is a load of information about this, but what I immediately understood was that the optimal discharge is apparently clear to yellow in colour, and if you have some between your index finger and your thumb and stretch it, it should resemble that of egg whites. It should stretch a few centimetres without breaking! Gross, I thought to myself, but here goes.

This became a daily check, in fact, multiple times per day. Now, if I get this egg white stuff paired with a smiley face, surely that means I am ovulating or soon going to ovulate. I still couldn't tell, sometimes it was watery, other times there was none! I would examine it and think about whether it's watery or stretchy, but I couldn't decide. Mind-boggled, I would Google images of ovulation discharge and, my God, some of the things you would see would frighten you! I didn't seem to have mucus like those pictures, and for that I was kind of happy because some pictures were really 'out there'. On top of all of that, I was flying through the tests, and they are really expensive. As for when I would go to buy them, I was petrified that I would run into someone I knew or some kids from school, and me with my arms full of tests in the queue.

In March 2022, my desperation to see those lines appear was growing. I was trying to hide it, but I was becoming obsessed with dates, charting my mucus, adding any twinge or pain I felt to the app, wondering if it was a sign of ovulation or not. I always get a pain mid-cycle, and I always thought it was my appendix or something; again, my knowledge was so limited. I learned from my new best friend, Dr. Google, that this was known as Mittelschmerz. A sharp, dull pain that lasted approximately a day for me. This is basically a sharp pain where the egg is about to burst its way out for ovulation. Now that I've figured that out, I thought, "Great, between the tests, mucus, and pains, I'll definitely know when to get busy."

I still didn't seem to get it right. March passed, and still no pink lines. A whole new level of desperation and self-blame began. This was real 'mind fuckery', as I refer to it. I couldn't figure it out. I hated when things got the better of me. I started to search, "How long before my period can I do a pregnancy test and get an accurate reading?" It didn't matter what it said online, I wanted to know before my dreaded period came because the thoughts of finding out again with pains and cramps to really remind you that you are not pregnant was a killer. That was it, I was hooked. I was going to buy pregnancy tests tomorrow and have them in the drawer for the next time I was within a day or two of getting my period to try to find out. I just didn't have the patience to wait.

I felt embarrassed about what I was doing, and I thought Mel would think I was mad. So, I secretly sneaked them into my bedside locker and didn't say anything. Day by day, I was still checking mucus, checking the app, and even putting in my water intake each day in sheer desperation. The app was constantly being opened, checked, and updated. It's all I thought about. The next thing that I learned was that sperm can live up to 4/5 days if the PH balance is correct and the consistency of mucus is correct. More things to worry about!

Let's talk lube...
So, it turns out that some lubricants can be acidic and create far from ideal conditions 'in there'. Now, I had to go and research safe lube to use. As always, everything I needed to know was searched in 'Mumsnet,' A platform where real people share issues of all sorts in life. It's not just about babies or fertility. I used to type a question in the search bar and follow it with 'Mumsnet' to get threads of information from real people. Notably, this should not be taken as medical advice, as it is literally just regular people having conversations. But it gave me food for thought and new topics to Google. I absolutely do not recommend it as the only source of information, as the people on that platform are not necessarily qualified or educated in these areas of expertise. This is where I heard about pre-seed, a highly recommended water-based lubricant that apparently helps sperm to reach their destination safely. There are very mixed reviews about it online, and I didn't buy it immediately because I thought some of the conversations about it were a little mad. I was sceptical, so I gave it a miss at this stage. But I couldn't believe I was searching online about lubricants. Desperate times, desperate measures, eh?

Chapter Five

Mothers' Day came about, and I yearned to be one. A mother. I felt so hard done by. A reminder that each year, many people dream of becoming a mother but know they may never get the chance, or that their chance has slipped away, perhaps more than once. So, be mindful of that.

April came and went, and still no pink lines. I cried lots and became really stressed about the situation. What the hell was I doing wrong? Was it because I drank two cups of coffee, or because I smoked a cigarette one night, or something else? It has to be my fault. I had words with myself, and told myself that I am not doing anything wrong and when the time is right, it will happen. I was trying to convince myself of that, but it didn't work. I kept digging and digging online, reading forums with other people's stories, again trying to find the solutions. The moment I woke in the mornings, I opened the app and thought about how I felt. Adding every minor feeling or sensation in my body, my water, checking mucus, checking predicted ovulation, and so on...the cycle continued day in day out, it's all I could think about. I was consumed.

Now, it was almost May, my birthday month. Could I ever be so lucky? Here we go again, checking, monitoring, and timing bedroom activities, which were beginning to feel more like a chore than for enjoyment. I relentlessly checked for those smiley faces and that egg white mucus of dreams! I can't say I ever really clearly identified both with confidence. I couldn't help myself; it was two days before my period was due. This was it. I was going to take a test in absolute hope. I just couldn't wait any longer. Once again defeated with a negative test. Devastation kicked in. I cried and cried in Mel's arms on the couch for the evening. The next day was a new start. I got on with things, but it was on my mind that this test might not be accurate. The next day was the date my period was due, and I was going to take another test.

    It was now the last Saturday in May. That afternoon, I said to Mel, "I just feel like I need to do another one." He looked at me with fear, fear that I would be so broken-hearted again for the remainder of the day, but he came and sat in the bedroom and waited with me. While we waited, we spoke about what we would do if it were negative again. He explained to me that he hated seeing me so disappointed, and he was worried about me. I promised that if the test was negative, I would move on, try to reset and stop testing and timing to see what would happen. I was so nervous. I counted down from three, and we looked at the test together.

    There it was, a very faint line. The very line that we had been waiting for. Immediately, we just looked at each other with caution and then sat in silence, staring at it. I mean, it was so faint that we held it against the light, the window, and waited a little longer, before turning the lights of our phones on it. The next question was, is this an accurate result? Is it an evaporation line? Is this it? It was so faint it was hard to be sure. We couldn't believe it. We hugged, smiled, laughed, kissed, and cried. This was the moment we hoped for, and we were in shock. My poor Mel had a major reality check. He was shaken. Mel's face resembled that of sheer panic. He went quiet, and the blood drained from his complexion. I watched as he held the test in his hand and stared at it. I stood back, my face in my hands, and said, "I can't believe it" about 1,000 times. The pure joy that consumed us was unbelievable. We agreed that I should wait another day or two and do another test to be sure it wasn't a false positive, and that we should try not to get too excited for fear that it was false or wrong. But I couldn't help myself. I went into overdrive. I took some pictures to try to capture the joy and shock from the moment. I still have them saved on my phone, and I look at them from time to time.

We went back to the kitchen and decided to have tea and sit and chat. I smiled from ear to ear. I remember lying on the couch as we chatted, and at one stage, I farted as I laughed. Mel just looked at me and my response was, "Oops, it's the baby, sorry"...I heard myself say those words, "It's the baby!" I thought I was hilarious and sure this was a great excuse now to get away with things. I rubbed my stomach, and Mel gave me a long hug and also rubbed my stomach. I couldn't believe that our baby was in there. Our future. We finally did it; I could breathe and relax a little. We were elated to say the least. We just couldn't believe it. Straight away, we discussed so many things, like the fear of being responsible for a child, how we would deal with situations, different traits from our upbringing that we wanted to carry forward with our little baby, and also what traits we did not want to carry forward. Talk about being in utter disbelief. Such a weird feeling. Already, Mel had become extra caring and protective. He spoiled me that day and told me to just relax. I spent the whole day on Google, of course, checking out symptoms of pregnancy and how can I identify early pregnancy. I searched the chances of a false positive pregnancy test, and how I could tell an evaporation line from a real line, and many, many other things. I spent the day on cloud nine. And on Google.

We got a text to say our friend was having a gathering for her 30th birthday. It was last-minute.com and just a small gathering in their house, if we wanted to come and join them. We wouldn't have missed it for the world; however, I was caught. How the hell was I going to go there and not drink or smoke a sneaky cigarette without giving it all away? It was too early to tell anyone, and I obviously wouldn't have taken any chances. I was working the next day in the airport, so that would be my get out of jail free card. And I wouldn't usually bother smoking a cigarette if I wasn't drinking. I would tell them I couldn't drink because I was driving very early the next morning. I remember standing in the kitchen chatting to some of the gang there, and all that was going through my head was don't touch your stomach, don't say you are pregnant, don't give it away. Mel glanced over at me every now and then, and we exchanged little smiles and winks. It felt so fun having a massive secret. I headed outside to sit with the girls and brought along my cup of tea that I had made inside. I probably totally gave it away by overcompensating, talking about how I had to drive in the morning.

We stayed a couple of hours, and when the alcohol was hitting them all at the party, we headed home. I was delighted, so elated, so happy and ready for bed for the first time as a pregnant person.

We talked and talked about scenarios and what if this and what if that, as we both drifted off to sleep, absolutely thrilled, both of us held my tummy with affection.

The next day, I was due to take some kids to Dublin Airport who were returning to Spain after a stay here. Can you remember the day the airport went buck-mad crazy after Covid? It was all over the news as the airport had dismissed all of the floor staff and as a result, the airport was not in control or being personed at all. There was a queue out the road, thousands of people missed flights, there was no staff, and it was just crazy. There were marquees outside to protect people from the weather as they queued socially distanced. Well, I was there that day. Mel tried to get me to cancel going and to try to get someone else to do it. He gave me a lecture that day before I left the house, "Drive slowly, be careful. If you are tired, just pull in. Make sure to eat. Don't lift bags. Don't get stressed, etc., etc." Basically, I had to promise to really mind myself.

I got to the airport, and you couldn't describe the mayhem that followed. It was insane. The queue wait time was about 5 hours long at best. People were angry, bags were lost, flights missed and cancelled.

I stood in a slow queue for about 2.5 hours before I called Mel, really upset. I didn't want to be standing there; I was afraid something would happen before I got to confirm everything with the doctor. I had to try to arrange rebooking flights with the agency that the kids travelled with, and try to console crying teenagers who were afraid that they would never get home. They were broken-hearted as they were just ready to go home and see their families. Some of them had been here for the full school year. I wanted to go home too, but I couldn't. Eventually, we got them sorted on flights and through security after about 7 hours. I still had to drive home, and I couldn't wait to get home and go to bed. I was wrecked. I had planned to call the doctor in the morning (Monday) and make an appointment to confirm that I was pregnant.

On Monday morning, I woke up with some pains, but thought nothing of it. It wasn't that bad; I assumed it was implantation after obsessive Google searches that morning. I went to school and started to teach my 9 am class. I set some work for the class and went out of the room to call the doctor to schedule an appointment for that day to confirm I was pregnant. I also decided to go to the bathroom while I was out of the room (bold, I know, leaving the class unattended).

There it was, I was bleeding. Initially, I didn't panic because I thought, "Oh, that can happen with implantation according to my morning research." I called the doctor and hid in the bathroom while on hold. All while in fear that my boss would realise I wasn't in the room, but what could I do? I explained the situation to the doctor's secretary, and the doctor rang me back straight away. I told her that I had what I think is a positive test, and I was planning to have it confirmed with her. She told me to go straight to the hospital's EPU (early pregnancy unit) and have things checked out. She was going to fax ahead so they would see me quickly. I started to panic. I was shaking and crying, my voice quivered as I tried to act cool and respond to her.

She reassured me that there might be nothing wrong, that sometimes women bleed in the early stages and not to worry. She said, "Go now, you have until 10:45 before they close for the day." I didn't know what to do. I was all over the place. Instant panic began, I could feel the adrenaline kick in, the shakes were astounding. The fear was totally taking over. But I also tried to talk myself into the idea that things could still be ok. I had to gather my thoughts; I dashed into the classroom and grabbed my things. I told the class (with tears in my eyes and a shaky voice) that something urgent had come up and I had to leave in a hurry and that I would have someone come sit with them and asked them to please do me a favour and be good while they waited.

I saw a colleague in her office, and I ran in and said, "I can't explain, but I have to go. Can you please sit with my class in the room. I have to go. It's an emergency." I also asked her who I should tell that I have to go (as I was running up the corridor). I ran to the other side of the campus and spoke to a member of management, but I didn't explain much. I was fighting back the tears, my lower lip was shaking, adrenaline was pumping through my body as I said, "I have to go, I can't say much right now, but it's an emergency and I have to go." I ran to my car and called Mel. I told him everything, and I said, "I'm on the way to the hospital now." He said he would meet me there, and I don't know what I was thinking, but I said, "No it's grand, I'll let you know if I need you, hopefully it's something simple like implantation bleeding. I'm sure it's ok."

I didn't let on how terrified I was.

He asked me several times if I was sure, to which I replied, "Yes," but I didn't mean it. My head was up my arse and, sure, I didn't want to be an inconvenience or for him to be down money in his wages if it wasn't necessary, that would have made me feel foolish.

I parked the car and ran inside; I was whispering embarrassingly to the reception area asking where is the Early Pregnancy Unit. I thought to myself (they know now, my secret is out, I'm pregnant, and something is wrong). I got to the reception desk in the EPU and gave them my name. They told me to sit in the waiting room down the hall. I sat in there and spoke to Mel again, he said, "I'll come up now sure, I'll be there soon." I replied with, "No need, stay at work. I'll ring you if I need anything. Sure, I could be sitting here for the day." Again, I felt like I better not make a big deal of this.

I had no idea what to expect, but I knew there would probably be an internal scan, and I had never had one before. As I sat in the waiting room, I looked at all of the other women waiting there and wondered were they in the same boat as me. I tried to gather myself and tell myself everything could still be ok. I was called into a room by a lovely, caring nurse. She asked me had I ever been there before and I said no.

She commenced explaining the process to me in simple language. I had to have blood tests done to see if there was evidence of the pregnancy hormone known as HCG. To the best of my memory, she said that if the HCG levels were 10 mIU/ml or above, it suggested pregnancy was indeed in place. It is expected that the HCG level will double every 2-3 days in early pregnancy. It turns out mine was at 15 mIU/ml. They rather see this over 25 mIU/mL but I was very early. They also did a test for progesterone.

Progesterone is critical in supporting a pregnancy because it thickens your uterine lining. This helps a fertilised egg grow into an embryo, and then into a living foetus. Progesterone levels continue to rise during pregnancy and help to maintain the pregnancy. High progesterone levels prevent your body from ovulating while you're pregnant. Levels that indicate pregnancy are approximately 10 to 44 ng/mL during the first trimester of pregnancy. Mine was at 22 ng/mL. So, there we go, finally, confirmation that I was pregnant, I wasn't imagining things, and I didn't dream it up. A relief to some degree.

Now I knew I could get pregnant. This then triggered the immense fear of losing this long-sought-after little life. I hardly had time to process that a baby was 'in there', but I had such a strong connection, desire, and love for this little baby that was only then the size of a dot! The nurse explained that I would have the bloods done, have an internal exam and then see a consultant. Then, two days later, I would come back and repeat the same pattern of tests to confirm if a pregnancy is developing or dwindling. She asked me if I had any pads with me. I didn't, as I wasn't expecting a period or bleeding, so I wasn't prepared.

She kindly handed me some pads and directed me to the bathroom to sort myself out. I was so embarrassed that she knew I was just sitting bleeding there in my underwear, but what could I do? It all had happened so fast. I had lined my underwear with tissue to save me from embarrassment in that sense, but I had to keep changing it regularly. Lesson learned.

The next step was an internal examination. I was not looking forward to this, despite having had smears done before and I don't particularly mind them. I was embarrassed because I was bleeding. I felt sorry for the radiographer carrying out the exam, and I apologised to her prior to the testing and said, "I'm sorry that I am bleeding; it's not very pleasant for you to have to do this." When I think back, what kind of a mentality did I have, and where did that come from? It wasn't my fault, and I couldn't help it.

She was so lovely and reassured me that it was she who should be apologising to me, and that I was in that situation, and that because it was so early, she would have to do a deep examination to ensure that there wasn't an ectopic pregnancy. I prepared for the exam, hopped up on the bed and covered my dignity with a sheet that was provided. While I waited for the exam to begin, I looked at the scanner machine and the probe they used, and I thought to myself, "Oh sweet holy God, is all of that going to go inside of me?" The radiographer took a condom, put it on the probe, added a generous topping of lubrication, and said, "Ok, are you ready to go?"

    I was utterly mortified to open my legs for the exam to begin. I was bleeding and felt unprepared in terms of cleaning myself up, but I didn't have a chance, and they wanted to see what was occurring. She made me feel so at ease. I took a deep breath and closed my eyes. I felt tears roll down my cheek as I fought hard not to cry. The radiographer was really supportive and was obviously so empathetic that I was in discomfort.

    It was uncomfortable mentally and physically. And then she said, "I am so sorry, but I'm going to have to go deeper. So, take a deep breath and slowly let it out." At that, she pushed slowly but with strength as she had to wriggle the equipment from side to side, to check the fallopian tubes for an ectopic pregnancy. If this were the case, and if left untreated, it could lead to serious infection. I moaned with the discomfort, squeezed my eyes closed even tighter, and grabbed onto the sheet on the bed with clenched fists. I eventually opened my eyes and gazed at the screen, foolishly thinking I would see some sign of the baby. I asked her, "Is there anything there?" Maybe I was delusional and clinging to hope that everything would be ok. How innocent was I? It was far too early to be able to see a baby. At most, I should have only expected to see a pregnancy sac. This would appear as a black circle on the scan. I could see nothing. The exam was over. The radiographer didn't say anything to me like, "Oh look, here is the baby." Instead, there was silence as she tidied away the equipment.

I asked her, "Is there anything there?' She told me that, "At the moment, there are no signs of anything. However, if it is as early as we think, there wouldn't necessarily be any sign yet anyway." She proceeded to say that one good thing is that I was not experiencing an ectopic pregnancy. I took that as a positive and tried to reassure myself that it could all still be ok.

I was told to go and wait in the waiting room to see the consultant. I waited in a room with other women. Some appeared to be in for a routine check, others had a worried look about them, and others were visibly in pain and emotional. I didn't know what to think or where to look. Such a plethora of emotions and body language in that one room. At this point, I really wished Mel were there. I was so vulnerable, lost, scared, and really needed support. It wasn't his fault, I literally told him to stay at work several times and, sure, he didn't know differently either.

About one hour passed, and I was the only one left in the waiting room. I was beginning to wonder if I would be seen or if I had been forgotten. Suddenly, a rather largely built man appeared in the room and asked if I was waiting to see a consultant, followed by asking me my name. He left, only to return and explain that he was actually the consultant.

For some reason, he had decided to check the waiting room himself, even though he'd been told everyone had already been seen and gone. Strange...

I entered the room and took a seat; there was a friendly nurse in the room also. He asked me why I was there that day, I explained and he then took time to check the charts and results and talk me through everything. He explained that I would come back on Wednesday and have all of the tests repeated, and that the levels will indicate what is happening.

He was comforting, caring, and told me to take it easy, to rest and put my feet up and to be kind to myself. He told me not to take pain relief for the cramps because at that point the bloods indicated a viable pregnancy. He advised me not to use tampons and to drink lots of fluids and explained that if there were signs of a developing baby in the scan on Wednesday, but the bloods indicated pregnancy loss with reduced HCG levels, that I would have to have a medical procedure known as a D&C. This is the removal of any tissue associated with a pregnancy as a precautionary measure to prevent infection. He told me to keep an eye out for large clots passing and to come back if I felt I was bleeding heavily or had severe pains.

I left and walked to the car. I called Mel and told him everything, and I cried so hard as I drove home alone. I couldn't wait to get home and have his arms around me. I felt immense sadness and had an outpouring of emotions when I got home. God love him, this was all new language to him, and he hadn't been there to witness what happened, so I'm pretty sure he didn't quite comprehend what I had experienced.

I had heard a lot of this language before from family and friends who had been pregnant or knew people who were pregnant, so at least I had a basic understanding as to what they were talking about. My God, that was a really horrible evening. I sat on the couch, exhausted from crying, distraught at the potential outcome. The joy was wiped clean, nowhere to be found as sheer sorrow crept in.

Chapter Six

I decided to go to school the next day. It was the last week of term, and I had a role as the exam aide. This meant that I was responsible for organising the state exams in our school that were due to start the following week. I still had some things to finish organising, including setting up some rooms and jobs to get done. I spoke to the same member of management that I had spoken to the day I left school and explained what was happening. They offered a genuinely kind response and asked me if I was sure I wanted to be there. They said they could finish organising things for the exams and offered to help. Me being me, a control freak, decided that, no, it was best if I did it because I knew it would be done right!

Going in would be a good distraction, and as well as that, I needed to get those last few things organised before Wednesday. I knew that if I got bad news on Wednesday, I wouldn't be able to go in and face people. I asked for permission to go in and do what I had to do for the exams, but not to teach classes that day. Kindly, this was facilitated. I'll never forget looking for one particular colleague who I needed to help me with a task.

That person was being funny and sarcastic that day, as always, but I wasn't able to take it. They were dragging things out, not saying if they would or wouldn't do the things

I needed help with. I lost it, I bawled crying and just said look, "If you only knew what was on my mind at the moment, can you help me or not because I am not able for this today?" They looked at me and just said, "Yes, I can." I said, "Good, thank you," and left. You could cut the tension with a knife.

I hid in the bathroom and sobbed. I had my head in my hands and was thinking to myself what the hell am I doing here and that I can't do it. I can't face people. I was mortified. There were a few people in the room at that time, and I just dropped my guard and showed them all my weakness. I cried for what seemed like no reason at all. I felt like an idiot, but I was also so angry at this person. On top of that, every bathroom trip was just another bleak reminder of what was potentially happening to my little baby.

I pulled myself together and went around the school with my plans for the examination centres, and continued to finish off whatever was needed to be completed in terms of tasks. During break time, I hid again, because I didn't want to see anyone. I was afraid I wouldn't be able to hold my emotions in.

The last bell of the day rang, and I decided to wait until the school was empty to do the last round of checks and ensure that everything was done. I had left word with management that one small job remained to be done if I wasn't in for the rest of the week. After that, I headed home again with my head hung low. I just had a feeling things weren't ok. I desperately wanted this baby, and it was so hard and frustrating to even get to this point.

That evening dragged; I spent hours with my friend, Dr. Google, searching for hope. I searched things like 'stories of women bleeding in early pregnancy but everything was still ok', and 'how to tell if I am losing a baby in early pregnancy'. Again, I cried and cried. I took a bath, but not too hot, because that doesn't help in early pregnancy. I went to bed to rest, but couldn't sleep. My eyes didn't dry up for even a minute. Mel was so caring. He really did all he could for me, ensuring I was fed (not that I had much of an appetite), comfortable, and covered me in blankets. He also offered his love and support, trying to reassure me. He was beyond brilliant to me, and hated to see me so upset. The time ticked by so slowly, I just needed to know now. The 'not knowing' was killing me. It was like slow mental and physical torture.

Every time I went to the bathroom and wiped myself, I examined the tissue. If something was going to pass, I didn't want to miss it. I didn't know what to expect in terms of blood loss; it was very heavy, and I felt very crampy, especially on Wednesday morning, compared to Monday when it all began. I was told to look out for blood clots, but nothing alarming or obvious passed. I didn't see any evidence of a baby or tissue. I had another delusional moment of reassuring myself that it could all be ok.

In the meantime, I had heard about this guy who is a healer and can help restore energy if you are unwell. I knew some people who had attended him when they were sick. He apparently had a connection with spirits and was a medium. All I wanted was someone to stop my mind from racing. It was exhausting. I had messaged him on Facebook on Monday evening, but I didn't hear anything back until Tuesday. He told me to come in on Wednesday at 5:30 pm. I had messaged him previously for another reason, but I never got a response, so I was delighted that he was going to see me so quickly. It made me think that he knew something.

Wednesday morning came. It was time to leave the house for the second round of tests in the hospital. Mel had taken the day off work to bring me; he was still mad at himself for not coming to the hospital on Monday despite me telling him I was fine and didn't need him to come.

It was a quiet journey interspersed with a few tears. When we arrived at the hospital, I knew exactly where to go this time, but I still found myself looking over my shoulder to see if I could recognise anyone before turning down the corridor with the massive sign for the EPU. I checked in at reception and sat in the waiting room once again. The nurse called me out and took my bloods; it would take an hour for the results. She didn't really talk about my situation; she spoke about general things in a nice, pleasant, and friendly tone. She wished me well and said she hoped everything worked out for me. The fact that she was being so nice broke down some of my walls.

I couldn't compose myself without my eyes filling up and my voice shaking. She rubbed my hand and told me to take a deep breath and face whatever comes with strength. I paused for a moment, took a deep breath, slowly let it out, and lifted my head to look at her. I dried my tears and gathered my things. I felt a little stronger again.

I headed out to Mel, who waited outside the door (the nurse's recommendations). When I opened the door, he was standing there, staring into my eyes, wondering if I knew anything else. He reached out his hand and pulled me in close for a hug. We stood there for a moment, and I told him what had been discussed. We then made our way back to the waiting room. The unit was quite full that day, but there were some empty seats at the back of the waiting area, so we sat in silence and held hands while tears continued to roll down my cheeks. I tried so hard to stop it; I didn't want people to know that this was happening to me. I didn't want strangers to see me cry. However, I couldn't help myself.

Next up was the internal scan, which I was dreading. The cramps were stronger and the bleeding was heavier. I had given Mel a detailed explanation of the equipment used, what I had to do, what the radiographer does and gave him a broad idea of what to expect. As we waited, another woman came into the waiting room with her friend. She was so distressed and in immense pain. She sobbed and moaned in pain. I felt so sorry for her, and then I realised, oh wait, I could be the same. I got the impression that she was losing her pregnancy. She leaned on her friend's shoulder and cried so hard. She rested against the doorframe with her shoulder and head to prop herself up. She was angry; she hit the door frame with a closed fist. I wasn't judging her, not even for one second. In fact, in that moment, I forgot about myself and gave great thought to her.

At that, Mel and I looked at each other. I broke down, I couldn't hold it in anymore. I tried to do it quietly so people wouldn't be looking at me. He grabbed me, put his arms around me, and held me close. I could feel him breathing heavily, and when I looked up at him, his eyes were full of tears too. It was horrendous. The fear, the cold sweaty palms, rocking forward and backwards, waiting to be called. I walked the corridor to make sure that I wouldn't be forgotten this time because I couldn't go another day without knowing what was happening.

Every time I walked back into the room, I knew people were staring at me. I hung my head low, not wanting to make eye contact with anyone and took my seat again. We recognised a girl in the waiting room, we have both seen her around the town regularly, but I don't know her. Herself and her partner were talking loudly outside the door. He was using a strong, argumentative tone, a tone of disappointment, but also annoyance. The girl said, "Oh well, guess that wasn't meant to happen." He walked ahead, up the corridor and left her standing behind. He turned and said, "Will you ever give me a baby, for God's sake!" She followed him up the corridor and said, "I'm sorry, we can try again; I'll try harder next time." As if it was her fault. He replied with, "Forget about it, there won't be a next time."

Mel and I looked at each other in shock. We were astonished and could not believe what happened. That man was an absolute prick. Instantly, I thought it was an abusive relationship. I couldn't believe he was so cold and unsupportive to her, and I knew what she had been going through, and he literally didn't give one shit about her. I know what I would be telling him if that was me. At that, finally, I was called for the scan.

We entered the room; the nurse was placing a new sheet and pad on the bed. I made sure that Mel could come in this time because I needed his support. The nurse asked me to remove the bottom half of my clothing, lie on the bed, cover myself with the sheet, and that they would knock and ask for permission to come in again. It seemed like forever until they came back, but it was probably just three minutes. The same radiographer was working. She approached slowly and said, "Ok, are you ready?" I said, "Yes." This time, I wasn't as embarrassed as I opened my legs. I looked at Mel and held his hand. I took a deep breath and said, "Ok, I am ready." The examination began.

I wasn't as tense this time because I thought I knew what to expect. It seemed to take a long time. I gazed at the screen, looking for a glimmer of hope, but I didn't see anything. Of course, from my previous Dr. Google searches, I had looked up scan images of a baby five or six weeks pregnant to know what to look out for if anything was to be seen on that screen. The examination was over. The room remained very quiet. I think I already knew what was coming, but I still clung on to a smidge of hope. The radiographer said, "I'll give the scan results to the consultant, and he will discuss the results with you." I asked her to tell me if she has seen any evidence of a remaining pregnancy. She was silent and stared at me for a moment, and asked, "How honest do you want me to be?"

I replied, saying, "Very honest. I am a straight-up person; I need to know and don't beat around the bush." She asked me if I was sure, and I replied yes. She paused and said, "Ok. From my initial reading of the scan, I can say that I do not believe that there is a pregnancy remaining. I do not see any pregnancy sac, but equally, I do not see any tissue in the fallopian tubes. It is my view that you are not experiencing an ectopic pregnancy. I'm sorry."

She then paused once more and said, "I believe that you have lost your baby due to a miscarriage."

I just looked at her and thanked her for her honesty. That was it...the last thing I wanted to hear. I don't really know how I felt in that moment. I was numb, confused, and really trying to process what was happening. She told me to take my time getting dressed, and she left the room. I looked at Mel and said, "That's it, it's gone." I broke down crying for a couple of minutes before dragging myself back to the waiting room. We sat in a daze, hardly speaking but holding each other. I tried my best to keep it together.

A lady then came into the room; she was smiling from ear to ear. She sat in the seat directly in front of us and called someone to tell them the good news. Her baby was ok. She sat there elated as she unravelled her baby scan pictures in delight. Rightly so, she should have been so relieved, and I am happy for her. But that hurt so much. Here we were receiving absolutely terrible news, sitting amongst people with the best news ever. I couldn't help but stare over her shoulder at her scan pictures and say to Mel, "It's not fair, will it ever happen for us?" She sat for a while, staring at her scan pictures before her lift arrived, then she left.

Some time passed, and we were called in to see the consultant. It was a different man than the last guy, and he didn't have a nurse with him. I observed that he didn't have an Irish accent, only because I had to really tune in to make sure I understood and heard everything he was saying.

He invited us into the room; he had my chart in his hand with the scan image attached to the cover. It nearly sickened me to see it because there was nothing there, another reminder that it was all ending. He began by asking me, "Why are you here today?" I scrunched my face and thought, "Well, can't you see my chart?" but I didn't say that. I replied and said, "Well, today we are here because I have been bleeding and I am pregnant. I had to have tests today to see if I am still pregnant." I happened to look at the computer screen, and I could see my name and three other files with my name on them. He opened the first page of the chart in his hand and appeared to skim-read it in silence. I assumed he was taking a moment to inform himself about the situation. Seems I was wrong.

He appeared to read and read; he then lifted his head and said, "I don't know why you are here. It seems that you are exaggerating a long cycle; you have your period, that's all." I was so puzzled; I scrunched my eyebrows and face and looked at him with confusion. I looked at Mel, and we were in total shock; we then questioned the pregnancy. I said, "Actually, no, I was here Monday and had the tests done, and my bloods indicated a pregnancy was existing." I proceeded to tell him that my HCG was 15 and progesterone was 4. He then looked at me puzzled, he paused and said, "Oh wait, let me check something on the computer." He hit the refresh button, and then he said, "Ah ha, oh yes, your results have just been updated this moment. Now I can see them."

    I knew this was just not correct because I had seen the screen when I entered the room. There was nothing different about it. He was trying to cover up the fact that he hadn't a clue what was happening. I said nothing, I let him continue. He took a moment and raised his head to look at me and said, "Oh yes. It seems you had a miscarriage. You are empty; there is nothing inside of you!" (while rubbing his stomach).

    The room went silent; those harrowing and haunting words burrowed their way deep into my soul. I was empty! How could someone, a professional, say such a thing in such a delicate moment?

    Mel and I stared at each other in disarray. Did he just say that? We were taken aback. What has just happened? There was an awkward feeling in the room; it felt horrible. The silence just continued as neither of us knew what to say, do, or ask. The consultant didn't have anything to add. He just said, "Ok, well that's it. Do you have any questions?'

    I just couldn't make sense of it. I didn't know how I was supposed to feel. My head was all over the place, confused, shocked, and getting more and more angry. Everything felt upside down, yet I was just expected to sit there, take it all in, and somehow come up with the 'right' questions. I didn't know what I was meant to ask. The only thing I could think of initially was, "Do I need a D&C?" He said, "No, I don't think so." Oh, how very reassuring was that...I don't THINK so! I could feel my blood beginning to boil; I was getting ferociously angry at the way he dealt with this consultation. Why would he deliver news such as this in that cold, callous way? I'm not going to lie; I immediately thought to myself, "You are a fucking dickhead! I can't believe you are meant to be a medical professional; you're clearly in the wrong job.'

He looked away, fiddling with the computer, which indicated to us that we were done. I stood up and said, "Have you any advice for me going forward?" He turned on the swivel chair, looked at me, and said, "Well, like what? What else do you want me to tell you?" I shook my head in disbelief and said, "Well, I don't know. What should I expect bleeding-wise or pain-wise? In the future, if I want to try again, is there anything I need to know?" I then said, "You are the so-called expert here, not me. I have never done this before."

His reply was short, "Take Nurofen if you have to, and expect bleeding like a period. It may be slightly heavier, and you can try again whenever you want. If you pass any clots larger than a two-euro coin, come back in case you get an infection."

Speechless (for the first time in my life), I didn't know what to say or do. I was absolutely furious, and I knew that if I stayed there for much longer, I would probably tell him a few harsh truths that he would not like to hear. But that wasn't why I was there. Instead, I said to Mel, "Come on we are leaving," I gathered my things and I almost took the door off the hinges with the bang I gave it as I left. What a fucking prick! That's all I could think about as I walked by him and left the room.

Chapter Seven

Outside the door, I lost it. I cried so hard I couldn't stand it anymore. I squatted to the floor with my head in my hands. Our little baby that we hardly even knew was gone. We had so many plans for this baby. We had it all discussed and planned. We laughed at things we would do to play pranks on the baby as they grew up, and we felt that we had such a connection already. This was our child, and it was gone. It was something we wanted so badly, and it had been taken away from us; it was something I couldn't control. That day, I was noted as 6 weeks and 5 days into the pregnancy. It hardly existed in the eyes of some people I know, but that didn't make it any easier for me or for Mel.

  I gathered myself, and I just wanted to go home. We walked to the car in silence, holding hands. When we got into the car again, I sobbed. It wasn't fair. What did I do wrong? The blame game began! Was it because I had a coffee? Was it because I ate some chocolate? Did I lift bags at the airport that were heavy? Did I cause this? Mel reassured me the entire way home. The pains got worse. I think it's because I finally stopped fighting my thoughts that something was wrong. I had to give in and admit it; I was physically losing my baby, and it was beyond my control. The emotional pain made it feel worse. We stopped in a town on the drive home, and I went to the pharmacy. All I was allowed to take was ibuprofen, and I knew we had none at home because we don't really take medicine for anything, ever!

My eyes were puffy and swollen, my nose was red, my head was bursting, and I just wanted the earth to swallow me up and to sleep. I was so tired. When I walked into the pharmacy, I met the lady that I had mentioned previously, she propped herself against the door and hit the door frame in anger. The same lady had been inconsolable an hour prior to this. She was laughing with her friend, and they were chatting. She said, "I'm just not going to tell him about it" (I assumed 'him' was a partner or husband). She said he doesn't know about all of the other ones, so I won't tell him about this one. I understood this to mean that she had many losses before this. I couldn't believe how she had changed from the woman I saw, completely distraught, not long before that. She and her friend shared a laugh and had discussed plans to go get some drink in the supermarket across the road. They were going to have some friends over to help distract themselves. I couldn't believe it. How can you be so ok with this? How can your emotions have vanished from what I saw an hour ago? Why the hell wouldn't you tell your partner? How could you hold it in like that?

I got what I needed and left the pharmacy to go home at long last. On the way, I called my GP and told her the results. She asked me to come see her the next day, so I made an appointment and hung up the phone.

We got home and we went inside. I just sat on the couch. Mel made tea, covered me in blankets, and told me to lie down and not move for the day and made sure that I didn't need anything else. My mind was racing. I sobbed with anger, consumed by questions I couldn't answer. Why had this happened? How would I know if it had already passed? Had

I missed it? What would it look like? What was I supposed to do with it? Would it be big enough to see? So, where did I turn to? Only Dr. Google yet again. I hesitated because I wasn't sure if I wanted to see images, but off I went typing into the search bar something like, "6 weeks and 5 days pregnant losing baby, what to expect?" Or things like, "6 weeks, 5 days miscarriage, what does it look like?" The images were horrendous. But I always want to know in advance. I felt like I was breaking the law and being disrespectful to other people's losses, but I needed to see what others had experienced to know what I was going to experience or see. I hadn't been prepared by the hospital for this. It was far from pleasant; I didn't look for long and then locked my phone again and tried to shake it off and tell myself I will know. I won't miss it.

  I dreaded every toilet visit because I didn't know what I might be faced with. That whole day, it seemed that dark red blood was coming out. No clots or anything sinister. As the evening continued, so did the cramps, tears, and rage. Then, I remembered I had made this appointment with the healer. I didn't want to move, but I decided to go because I was desperate for anything to help me to be at ease. I didn't know what to expect. Mel drove me there, parked outside, and I went in. I was greeted by this man (the healer) and his wife, who was at reception. He invited me into this bare room with just two chairs and a little table beside the chair I was going to sit at. I noticed a box of tissues and a glass of water. He was a nice man, fairly comforting. We sat and just had some general chit-chat for a while. I thought it was odd; he seemed to have some weird twitch or something. He would look at me as we were chatting, and then it was like his head turned to the side really quickly, like he was following something moving with his head. I was kind of freaked out, but we carried on.

Then he said to me, "Oh my God. There is a lot going on around you." I was puzzled, I said, "What?" Then he said, "There is a loss here, I see a little baby." That was it; I lost control and began to cry. He asked me, "Did you recently have a loss?" I, a bit astonished, said, "Yes. Just today it was confirmed." He asked if I knew if it was a girl or a boy and I said no, it was too soon to know. He said he could tell me if I wanted. I thought about it for a second, and I really wasn't sure if I needed to know that because I thought it might add to the emotions if I knew who was in there, if I knew what I missed out on. But of course, I nodded yes. He said it was a little boy. I couldn't contain my sorrow. It just flowed. To think this little baby had an identity, it made its short existence so very real. He reassured me that this little boy just knew he wasn't going to make it, and he left before I could get too attached to lessen the heartache for us. He told me that this little boy said that he had never felt love like it before, and he was so happy that I was his mammy.

He told me that this little baby will always be with me and is a part of me now, that he knew he was so very loved already and was sad that he couldn't make it to be with us in person, in life. I was so sad...I didn't know if any of this was true or not, but do you know what, it gave me some strange feeling of communication or closeness with this little baby, my little baby, our little boy.

We talked about lots of other bits and bobs, but then he told me a bit more about himself. He told me that he always knew he was different from a very young age. He said he sees colours, not people. He referred to me as having a deep connection with the spiritual world, only I can't see it because I don't know how. I thought he was mad. As far as I was concerned, I was one of the least spiritual people out there. In fact, I was a real sceptic but I sought him out simply to give anything a go to help me to heal. Some of the advice he gave me was stone mad when I think about it. He told me to drink nettle soup, eat raw beetroot, and buy a hula-hoop and use it...a hula-hoop. I thought to myself, "What the hell do I want a hula-hoop for, ya mad yolk." He then went on to tell me that the movement used for hula hooping would help clear any blockages in the fertility area. Ah sure, in my desperation, sure as shite, that was it...I was going to turn into a hula-hooping queen.

  Afterwards, I sat in the car with Mel and told him most of the stuff on the way home. When we arrived, I told Mel that he had said it was a little boy, and I burst into tears again. We hugged, and I cried and cried more. My little boy is gone, and I couldn't protect him or control things. This ignited a severe battle in my head again about what I did wrong. Why was I a failure? What did I do to deserve this pain? Is it a punishment? Was I not meant to have a baby? Off my head went into a spin once again; meanwhile, all I could hear were the words the doctor used over and over, "You are empty, there is nothing inside." Jesus, if I could have got my hands on him at that point, God knows what I would have done to him. The evening came to a close. I was absolutely shattered, my face was swollen from crying, and my nose was red raw. I must have used three rolls of toilet roll that day for the tears and snots.

  I went to get ready for bed and had to face the toilet visit one last time before climbing into bed. Would this be it? Would I see something? I sat and braced myself for the wipe and check. There was nothing bar the expected blood. My mind tried to trick me into thinking, ok, well, no sign of anything yet, does this mean I could still possibly be pregnant? They could be wrong? I brushed my teeth and looked in the mirror. Delusional thoughts entered my mind. Ok, well maybe if the baby is still in there, it could be ok, couldn't it? Let's see what tomorrow brings. I quickly fell asleep because I was exhausted from being so upset.

Chapter Eight

I woke up Thursday morning, and I felt like shit. My head was banging, the cramps were progressing, and I was just so heavy and sad. I contacted work to tell them I wouldn't be in for the rest of the week and that I would be ready for the exams the following week. It was a slow morning and I took to the couch again in my pyjamas. I wasn't moving for the day. I just needed to rest and look after myself now. I cried a lot less during the day and sat in a dead stare, just thinking. I hardly really spoke. Mel took the day off to be with me and to look after me again. I was up and down to the bathroom quite a bit, but otherwise I was generally feeling ok until later that evening.

I went to the bathroom; I did the usual 'brace yourself', took a deep breath, and checked the tissue. And there it was. I couldn't believe it. It was so small and resembled a grain of rice in a half-moon shape. It stood out like a sore thumb despite it being so, so small. There it was, there he was...My little boy.

I'm not going to lie; I had no idea what to do with it. I cried from the pit of my stomach this time. I could finally see it; although it didn't look like a baby because it was so early on, it was the start of what was meant to be our family. I held the tissue in my hand and stared at it as I was still sitting on the toilet. I cried so hard I could hardly breathe. What do I do? Do I show Mel? Do I not? Do I keep it? Do I flush it? Nobody told me what I am meant to do with it. I felt that flushing it was, perhaps, uncaring, the wrong thing to do. How could I flush my baby away? It felt abusive...I didn't know what it was, but it felt wrong. I then thought, "Am I meant to bury it?" And if so, where? And in what? I do not know why I chose not to show Mel or at least give him the choice. I felt that he might be grossed out by it and feel that he would have to look at it, even if he didn't want to. I felt like I'm the woman here and I am meant to know what to do with this, and that I needed to deal with it. I thought it wouldn't be fair to show him; it was probably not for him to see (old traditional voices entered the building). I went to Dr. Google again and typed in something like, "What do I do with tissue from early miscarriage at home." Most of the answers were to flush the tissue as normal.

Suddenly, my thoughts changed, I couldn't look at it anymore, I was angry and upset. I just needed it gone, and maybe that would put an end to the horrible feelings that I was experiencing. I needed to make a decision, and I had to do it fast.

As I gazed intently at my baby boy before me, a tide of emotions surged through me. I felt small, alone, and utterly insignificant. Suddenly, these waves of emotion crashed against me, relentless and overwhelming, dragging me under and threatening to pull me beneath their weight. I panicked, I felt anxious. I looked at him one last time and sobbed. I tried to speak, but all I could manage to say was, "I am so sorry." Overwhelmed with guilt, I added, "I don't know what I'm meant to do, but I love you." With that, I flushed the toilet. The very second I did, the only emotion I could feel was regret. What kind of a bitch was I to have done that? What sort of mother would I have been if I could do that to my own baby, who was so small? I hated myself for what I had done, and I couldn't face up to it for a long time. I compartmentalised and blocked it out as best, and for as long as I could. However, I couldn't get that image of when I first saw him out of my head. I can still see him as clearly as I sit here and type now. I stayed in the bathroom for a few minutes; I crouched down, resting my head on the toilet seat, and cried. What did I do, I thought to myself. I'll never forgive myself.

I eventually shook myself off and went back to the living room. Mel asked me if I was ok, and I just said, "Yeah, I think some stuff might have come out," but I didn't go into it any further. I couldn't talk about it. I had to get the image out of my head. I had to turn cold and try to forget what just happened. We tried to carry on as normal as possible while also allowing ourselves to talk about it and feel whatever we needed to feel. Still, the heaviness of the sadness was very hard to navigate. It was time to tell my family because it was eating me alive. I needed to keep talking about it and telling this story because it was really shit, and I knew so many others had gone through it or similar.

Song: Beyoncé – Heaven (couldn't wait for you).

This song resonated so much. It's a song Beyoncé wrote for her uncle when he passed away. Because of this, not all of the lyrics were totally relevant to me, but this song still touched my soul, especially the chorus. I listened to it and tried to sing along many times, but I couldn't as my throat tightened up trying to hold back the tears. It's a beautiful song and melody. Now, I can listen to it and I still shed a tear, but I can try to sing along. I find that I listen to it on those days that the little baby is really on my mind. There is something touching about a song when it hits you and triggers an emotional response. This isn't the case for everyone, and some people will never understand that.

This was a time in my life when I was extremely vulnerable. The thought of going home to tell Mam and Dad was awful. I hated letting my guard down, I didn't want to appear weak. I never really spoke to my parents about anything personal; I just didn't feel that kind of connection with them. To be fair, they were always there if I needed anything, and they made that clear to us growing up. I did my own thing; I was Miss Independent from a young age. I went over to the house on my own and went inside. I didn't know what I was going to say or how I was going to say it, but I had to get it out. I took some deep breaths and told myself not to burst out crying. Try to keep strong. I walked inside and chatted for a second. I was filling the kettle and I just said, "So, I've something to tell you: I lost a little baby."

I was in convulsions, crying before I even finished the word 'baby'. I hadn't said it out loud before this, and that hurt. I was doubled over the kitchen counter, sobbing, and dad gave me the biggest hug, and he just held me as I sobbed.

When I finally lifted my head, I could see his eyes were also filled with glassy tears. Mam, who has mobility issues, understandably didn't come to give me a hug. She was quiet for a few minutes and then said to me, "Oh dear, these things happen." I know that this wasn't said to intentionally hurt me or with any bad malice intended whatsoever, but I was just lost for words at the response.

To be fair, mam did get up soon after when she was going to another room and did offer her arm around me. And I needed it. I know this is a horrible situation, and people don't know what to say, but I thought it would be the one place where I could be guaranteed sensitivity, softness, support, and understanding. What felt like the biggest weight on my shoulders ever was passed off quite blasé, with little or no significance really. It just felt like, "Oh well. I'm sure you'll get over it. It'll be fine." To add to this, they had no idea of the mental load I had been carrying in trying to get pregnant in the first place.

I remember leaving the house and being so angry. I received a response, but not the response I desired, hoped for, or expected. Again, I know this wasn't the intention; don't get me wrong, they were and still are, great parents to me and my siblings, and we had a very good life, and for that I am very grateful. I am a softie at the core, and I just needed a little more tenderness at this time. I was often told that I was very sensitive when growing up, which to me was basically a polite way to say stop whinging and get over it. I was annoyed that I had let my guard down, and I didn't feel any comfort when leaving. I felt let down and on my own to deal with my emotions. Why did I bother?

Following on from that, I didn't get one call or message from my parents asking me if I was ok, which really made me feel foolish for expecting more emotional support when I really needed it and, when I sought it out.

After that, we then told some siblings and family members on both sides of the family. This dark cloud was no stranger, as we all know someone who has experienced this kind of loss. The initial response was much warmer and compassionate, to be fair. They all extended their support and sorrow, and offered listening ears. That is what I needed anyway. Mel didn't really talk about it with others, but he doesn't do personal conversations with others beyond me anyway. It was really me that needed the support, in this way, at this time.

After some time, I did tell a very small circle of friends because I needed to talk about it, and cry it out. That's how I deal with things. I suppose it's seeking validation for my feelings, and I always want to know what they would think, feel, or do in that situation, too. To be honest, I think I needed some sympathy and empathy as well. To the best of my knowledge, nobody in this circle had gone through this before.

With this in mind, when I did tell them, the response was minimal. I think the reason for this is that they didn't know quite what to say or how they could help in a practical way. I needed someone to ask me if I was ok. I needed acknowledgement that I was allowed to feel the way I did. That I had reason to feel so shitty and sad.

That I had reason to grieve for this little life we lost, and that it was ok to want to continue to talk about it when I needed to.

Instead, I felt very lonely and unimportant. Apart from the very few who did check in on us (which I could count on one hand), we were very much left to our own devices, and it felt deeply lonely. It almost felt as if we didn't have the entitlement to feel sad for some little 'thing' that wasn't really a baby yet in some people's eyes. I won't lie, I felt like slapping some people for their responses saying things like; "Ah sure, it could be worse if you were further on" or "Sure, no harm" or, "What's for you won't pass you," "It was very early, wasn't it?" and "Ye can try again." I felt like saying, "I am trying here, trying not to slap you in the face."

One major hurdle for me personally was the fact that the world around me was moving on. I was stuck in this haze of intrusive thoughts and self-pity. I was still seeking the support and the answers that I desperately needed, and I couldn't get relief from overthinking. I decided that I needed to park my feelings for a while and try to get on with the exams in school. I knew that the following September, I was due to have shoulder surgery, and I would be off for 6-8 weeks. I said to myself there and then that I would wait until then to let it all register. I just couldn't handle it at that time. I needed to wait until the middle of September and hold things together until then.

Each day passed, my mood was sombre, and I felt quite dull in myself. I threw myself into the exams and used that as a welcome distraction. I was busy, I needed that. As the exams settled into a rhythm and everyone knew what was happening, my days became quieter. I spent a lot of time on my own. I kept thinking about how not everyone is as gobby as me, or may not have the confidence or knowledge to ask questions.

I thought about all of the women who may have been shamed into thinking their pregnancy loss was an 'exaggerated cycle' and made to feel foolish. I also remember thinking about all of the women who may have been misled into thinking this and how they may not have gone to the hospital again if the same thing happened. This was the moment that I decided I needed to do something about the lack of follow-up. I wasn't happy, and that consultant needed to be reminded that he wouldn't get away with his non-existent bedside manner and unsympathetic practice with everyone. I now had a major bone to pick with him.

I sat and thought about it, and after speaking with another close friend of mine, who also had experiences of losses before (in another hospital), I discovered that the treatment I had received was in total contrast to her experiences. Not to mention that the aftercare was also spectacular in this other hospital. I decided I was making a formal complaint to the HSE about the consultant who had dealt with me. I finally had some use for the research and writing skills that I had developed in my five years of college, and I was simply going to use my brains.

I jotted down my main points and thought about the structure. I opened the HSE website, the hospital website, as well as the EPU information, and then investigated and read through every policy related to patient care, well-being, pregnancy loss, consultant practice, and more. I spoke to someone that I knew who worked within the HSE and asked them, "Who should I write to?" And, "Who will actually read this?"

I was given two names, but I decided to go further than that. I sent a letter to every head of every Department within the particular hospital and the majority of the board members. I also sent it to some of the head honchos in the HSE itself. I needed this to be heard!

It was imperative for me that I would begin the letter with the statement that I am not seeking compensation of any sort, I am merely expressing my concern for others at what I perceived to be a lack of adequate care and empathy provided by a consultant in a very sensitive situation and that I was expecting communication about the same. I wrote a very detailed account about what happened. I was able to pull out points and quotations from many HSE policies and guidelines, highlighting the perceived failures of the hospital in achieving those aims or policy guidelines during the duration of my care. I wanted to hit him and all of the readers where it hurt, so I closed off the letter by stating that I hope the consultant's mother, sister, wife, or daughter never has to encounter such heartless and unprofessional ignorance in their lives, especially at a time of such fragility and vulnerability.

I had the letter proofread by someone who worked for the HSE. I know it wasn't as professionally written as it might have been because I had so much emotion in there, too. But it felt good to finally write it and send it. A couple of weeks passed, and I got a call from a member of management. She was very kind and apologetic and instantly apologised on behalf of the entire team. I stopped her there and told her that everyone else was remarkable; it was just that one individual that I had an issue with.

Anyway, after some time, she started spluttering and, in the most roundabout way, asked if I could identify if the doctor was Irish or not. She seemed to be afraid to ask directly, I believe, in case it might appear to be racist or impolite, but I said to her, "If you are asking me if the doctor was foreign or not, the answer is most probably yes. He certainly was not originally from Ireland as he hadn't a trace of an Irish accent." She said, "Oh, I wasn't wondering about his nationality at all, it's just we couldn't make out the signature to know which of the consultants was on the case."

In my mind, I found that odd because I was sure there were only two consultants working that day. So, it can't have been too hard to find out. Surely, there was a roster somewhere that could have been checked. Anyway, she reassured me that it was being taken very seriously and that it would be part of some very important meeting in the coming two weeks and that they would communicate with me further after that.

Chapter Nine

Summer was passing on by, the exams were finished, and I was helping out a local company in my spare time to keep myself busy. I carried on regardless, I worked long, late days and tried to just move on. I knew I was just pushing it back deeper and deeper into the back of my head until I was ready to commit to dealing with it. I knew it was bubbling up inside of me, and I just had to hold tight for another few weeks.

One day, I opened the post box and there was a letter marked with the HSE symbol. My stomach dropped as my mind went into overdrive, wondering what it was going to say. I brought it inside, put it on the kitchen island, and just looked at it for a few minutes before I opened it. I needed to be in the right frame of mind.

The letter stated that the issue had been raised with the consultant obstetrician/gynaecologist, along with other post holders and members of management in this field. They named the doctor and reassured me that the issue had been raised with him as well. One of the paragraphs was what I shall term an attempt at an apology that went something like this…

The letter included an acknowledgement of the lack of empathy; it confirmed that a review of the file and results indicated that, yes, there was a pregnancy. This was followed by what Mel and I felt was a lame apology on the doctor's behalf, oh, and reassurance that the doctor would be more cognisant going forward. In my mind I was thinking, "Oh yeah, I'm sure he will alright." It reassured me that they had implemented new policies to ensure a nurse is present with a doctor at all times when delivering bad news. They also claimed that every doctor coming into the unit will be reminded to speak to people with dignity and clear communication at all times. Blah, blah, blah...If you ask me, nurses don't get nearly enough credit and also have to deal with the sometimes-inflated egos of consultants in their day-to-day work. This response was not going to change my situation; however, it might change the way some other people are treated, people who are fearful to speak up or ask questions. That was the end of that. I just wanted a 'call out' for terrible bedside manner. It gave me some sense of relief that I got to have my side heard. Whether the response was generic or genuine, I'll never know, but I'm going to take it as a sign that I was heard and it was noted.

Chapter Ten

So, after some time had passed since losing the pregnancy, we slowly started shifting our mindset to trying again. It was hard; it felt like we were almost ignoring the poor little soul that still hadn't left my mind for one second. Nothing had happened in August, so we spoke and I did some research.

I became obsessed with listening to podcasts and scrolling through Instagram for the answers...AOK Nutrition taught me a lot about women's health and hormones. I decided to go back to basics and learn about my cycle. One of the most profound moments was when I discovered that there are really only a short number of days in the month when you can get pregnant...WHO KNEW!!!! Again, if I had paid attention or shown any interest in science and biology in school, I might have known more about this. I found myself being led down many roads; watching videos, reading comments, and taking notes from podcasts. It's kind of embarrassing admitting I didn't have a clue about this stuff and the details behind getting pregnant, but I am sure that I am not the only one. That's why I am sharing my story.

Anyway, the videos were detailed but in easy-to-understand language. I had heard women before talking about getting bloods done to check hormones on day 21 of their cycle. I thought to myself, "Yeah, great. Sure, I'll get that done and see if there is anything outstanding or out of order going on in there that means I can't support pregnancy." And then AOK Nutrition had a video reaffirming the point that the 21-day hormone bloods are not an accurate way of testing because not everyone has this perfect 28-day cycle. Apparently, this is the ideal cycle to have.

Some women have a 36-day cycle or longer; and therefore, the hormonal activities that you would expect to see in a normal cycle at 21-days aren't going to be accurate for those women. It's basically a very generic test.

I continued to track my days. I wanted to get this right. I rang my GP's office and asked for an appointment in relation to my hormones and bloods, and the secretary said, "Come in tomorrow." I replied, "No, it has to be on a certain day, that is the problem." I got the vibe she was like, "Oh right grand, whatever..." but I gave her the date and asked for a time to come in. That was that sorted.

Day 21 came, and I was excited because to me, I was taking another step closer to finding out if things were functioning correctly. I went in and spoke to the GP and told her about the loss. She was very sympathetic, caring, and she listened. She acknowledged that it was ok for me to grieve and to feel that this little baby mattered. She spent a good bit of time with me and was really conscious and aware of the sense of loss and my vulnerable state. This was a first. Before this, I felt that I couldn't be stuck on these feelings; it was like people expected you just to brush yourself off and carry on. "Sure, don't be talking about it, it's gone and sure, it was very early anyway." It really felt unimportant when I tried to talk to others about it.

We did the bloods, and I asked her if the 21-day test is accurate, and she said, "Yeah, of course it is." I was thinking back to all of the information that AOK Nutrition had posted, and I started to question it. I gave the example of someone with a longer cycle or a shorter cycle and asked if it was accurate for them. I was met with hesitation until I kept asking and digging and then the doctor agreed that there was a discrepancy and potential inaccuracy. I was shocked, so many women are being misled about cycles and testing. She asked where I was getting my information from, and I told her. She comforted me once again with gentle words of reassurance and spoke to me about stress and how that can impact chances of getting pregnant. She spoke about society today being in such a hurry, always after the next thing and the result being that the body is unable to switch off into its standby mode. It's always in fight or flight mode. She told me to work on my stress levels and look after myself.

    I needed to start a bunch of new supplements to complement the prenatal supplements I was taking. I continued taking Pregnacare pre-pregnancy vitamins, Omega 3 fish oils, CoQ10, zinc, and a probiotic called Merlak. I wanted to be in tip-top shape. I was back in the gym and trying to get my energy back up. My mind was still quite negative despite me trying to convince myself otherwise.

Chapter Eleven

I wanted to do something to remember our lost soul. I didn't know quite what to do because I am as far from being creative as they get. We talked about planting a tree, and we found a vibrant one we liked with bright red leaves. It was a Japanese red leaf maple. It turns out that it wouldn't have thrived where we lived, according to the garden centres that I called, so we got another tree. I had it delivered, and I planted it. It was a little therapy for me. Mind you, we both laughed because, honestly, I'm better at killing flowers and plants rather than keeping them alive. I go out there sometimes and just linger about if my head is all over the place.

We picked a spot with a good view and imagined ourselves in the future with a child or children sitting under the tree on a sunny day. We talked about a swing set and making a little bench for under the tree. Although at the rate it is growing, it might be a very long time before it can shelter anyone from the sun. I'll probably be gone to the afterlife by then!

In the meantime, we were invited to go on a night out. The gym we go to has nights out and we usually do a bus tour to local pubs. Let's just say, they are mighty craic (for my international readers, that means good fun). I knew this was coming up, and I knew we needed to blow off some steam, but I was so afraid of how I might react with alcohol. I wanted to go out for Mel's sake. I was so gloomy; it must have been hard for him to be around that low energy all of the time.

I hummed and hawed over and over again, and then I said, "To hell with it. Let's go out and try to have some fun for once." I asked Mel to keep an eye on me, and if he noticed me getting very drunk or looking like I was going to get upset, to just get me out of there. I didn't want to have deep conversations with anyone either while drinking, as it is not a time, or place, for them to have to listen to me either. I got dressed up and we headed off. I wanted to let my hair down, but equally, I didn't want to ruin any chances of getting pregnant. Talk about a balancing act. A constant mind game.

Very often, I put things on hold, like meeting friends or going on work nights out, and so much more, because I was trying to create the perfect environment for pregnancy to happen. I really did become fairly secluded.

And so, it began. I could feel the alcohol hitting me, and I couldn't resist having a few more to make my thoughts go away. I drank shots with the girls, and then we were dancing as a large group. The whole group was there. I remember the awards were being given out, and I just felt the heaviness drag me down. I felt the drink hitting me hard, and I started to cry. I went outside and tried to get Mel on the phone. I can't remember who I sent in to get him, but he came out to me and arranged for one of the lads to leave us home. Thankfully, this pub was only two minutes from the house, and this guy didn't drink. I was crying in the front seat of the car and had my fill of drink. I could hardly get out of the car at the house. I thanked the guy who left us home, and then Mel had to help me inside. I was hardly fit to put one foot in front of the other, and I was just so tired. I apologised so many times for ending Mel's night too.

I needed him so much in that moment. I just needed to sleep it off and hope to God I didn't say anything too dark to anyone who was there. I chose not to think about that and to not allow the fear to creep in. I chose to believe that I just got out of there at the right time and didn't make a fool of myself...but who knows! I just may have. To make matters worse, when we came home, I had to have a good cry and then, of course, came the vomit. Too much information, I know, but, hey. Needless to say, we had a very slow start the next morning, and I felt really guilty for ending Mel's night early. I was right to be nervous about going drinking when things were so raw for me. Lesson learned.

We had booked our honeymoon for the end of July and early August. The timing couldn't have been better. We couldn't wait for the break. Ten glorious nights away from all of the reminders at the 5-star W Hotel on the Palm in Dubai. To hell with Covid, which had stopped us from going too far until that stage. It was a great break from everything. Such a class place to visit. The glamour, the lavish lifestyle, was just what we needed to try to relax and unwind again. It felt like a total reset. We had long, lazy pool days and (a few!) cocktails; I had a spa day, trips to the desert, shopping, sightseeing, and all of the rest that comes with the territory. We had plenty of very fancy meals too. Such a fun place to visit, and it did us the world of good.

We had a dog called Rocco, a beautiful corgi. He had a companion called Nemo who died in the first part of the Covid lockdown, at seventeen years old. My shadow! We had been talking about getting another companion for Rocco for a while, and on the last day in Dubai, we found her online by chance while watching the last sunset of our trip...another little corgi who had an adorable charm as the top of her ear had been nipped off by her sibling. It was good timing; I would be home for a few weeks post-shoulder operation to train her and make sure they got on together.

We went to visit her, the mother, and the father in the house a day or two later. She was the full 8 weeks old, but the family wanted to keep her with the mother another week, so we had to wait, but she was so cute. We loved her instantly. She had a bold temperament, was mad as a hatter, and was full of attitude. She would certainly fit in. She was a very welcome distraction, who also tested my patience, let me tell you. We named her Willo. She has been no more than a few feet away from me for this entire process.

I decided to book myself in with a fertility specialist to see if there was anything in particular that could make conception a little easier and to see if there was anything obvious that may have caused the miscarriage. I was so afraid that I had left it too late, and my body didn't want to get pregnant at the age of 36. I had heard so much about the so-called geriatric mothers (anyone over the age of 35). I was officially an 'auld one!' I wanted to give us the best chance at making this happen, and I wanted to try and save ourselves the time and heartache by checking if there was anything wrong. I really wanted to ensure a smoother process this time.

We had booked an appointment for the week after the honeymoon. Of course, this was a private appointment, and it was expensive. But at this stage, we didn't care.

In the meantime, I was researching things like IUI (Intrauterine Insemination) and IVF (In Vitro Fertilisation). Some may say I was getting way ahead of myself, but I felt under so much time pressure from the ticking clock. It's almost like it was just expected for us to be pregnant too after just getting married, you know well that eyes are watching and waiting. I had so many people still asking me, "Do you think you would like to have kids?" I used to just smile and say, "Ah who knows, what will be will be." Inside, I would be devastated and thinking, "If they only knew how each day is such a challenge right now."

Chapter Twelve

At long last, the day of the appointment with the fertility specialist had finally come about in August 2022. The drive to Dublin seemed to take forever. We got there and couldn't get parking close to the hospital, but we had allowed lots of time. We walked in the front door and had to give our details due to Covid traceability and answer a questionnaire. They provided us each with a mask, and in we went. I had to go to the bathroom first. I asked for directions and went in. The toilet was beside what appeared to be a clinic waiting room. There were many very pregnant ladies around. I went into the cubicle, and there was a lot of blood in there. All I could think of was that some poor lady was bleeding, and I hoped that it was because she was in expected labour and not experiencing a miscarriage.

    This place had people here that were experiencing God knows what. I waited to use the other cubicle and went back out to Mel. We headed towards the general direction of the consultant, and met a man carrying a car seat with a very small baby. I wondered where the mother was. We talked, and I said, "God, I wonder what is wrong with her. I hope he didn't lose a partner." We met another couple walking out, smiling from ear to ear as they walked very slowly, carrying their bundle of joy to the car. I just thought it was absolutely fabulous. We both looked at each other, and I said,

"Hopefully that can be us someday." I smiled in hope and in awe of the cuteness, but I was also very sad to think that we may never get to walk out the door with our very own. My mind went straight back to the fact that I should be pregnant and getting ready to meet our little baby.

After meeting many people and chatting amongst ourselves as we wondered what their story was, we got to the consultants' waiting area. I checked in and took a seat. We waited nervously. I wasn't that excited about the scan. I hoped that nothing would be wrong, yet feared the opposite. I thought about all sorts of scenarios; what would I do if he told me I needed surgery, or if I couldn't get pregnant, or if he found a growth or something scary in the internal scan? I just didn't know what to expect, and I was shaking and breathing very heavily. I was very anxious as we waited to be seen by the consultant.

My name was called; I scrambled to gather my coat and bag, and we went in, exchanging a deep breath and a nervous glance. We were welcomed in, sat down, and the Dr said, "Hello." We had some small talk and then we got to business. The doctor asked me a series of questions about my health, my cycle, any experience with pregnancy or loss, family history, and, of course, all of the details about the miscarriage.

All along, it had been referred to as a miscarriage, and then out of nowhere, he said to me, "We call this a chemical pregnancy." I looked at him, confused. He said, "Yes, it's where a pregnancy doesn't quite get a chance to develop for some reason or another, and it is expelled at a very early stage. There is an imbalance or something amiss. It's nature's way. If it seems that a baby might struggle or may not make it, nature knows this, and it does its own thing." I thought to myself that this term 'chemical pregnancy' seemed dismissive. It kind of felt like there was nothing there to lose in the first place, by the way he described it, but for me, there was certainly something there. I felt like a shrinking violet, embarrassed once again for having such deep feelings about this 'chemical pregnancy'. It felt like it didn't even include a human. It was made up.

    He told me he would do a full assessment. I presented the blood test results from the test that I had done, and he said it all looked fine, that the markers were all good. The date of the appointment had been lined up with the pending ovulation or the approximate day that ovulation was expected to happen. He asked me to hop up on the table, and he told me all about the internal scan that he would do and what he was going to look at. I was nervous for obvious reasons, but not as shy as before. I was afraid I didn't have the dates right and that I wouldn't be near ovulation. He inserted the probe, and within a minute, he said, "Everything I am seeing in here is textbook, absolutely perfect." Talk about having such a sense of pride of my 'lady bits.'

    He mentioned the uterine lining, egg follicles, tubes, and whatnot. He turned the screen around to face me and asked me if I knew when I was ovulating. I told him I'm not sure of the exact day, but I do get a pain for about 12 hours or so, which I think lines up with my ovulation day. He asked me if I knew which side I was due to ovulate on. I said yes, I always knew from the pain which side was releasing an egg. It was only recently that I put two and two together and established that these were ovulation pains. They can be quite sore at times, and I often wondered if my appendix was giving bother. He said to me that there was an egg literally ready to come out, that it would be out in the next 12 hours or so and joked that now this is a great time to get busy. We all laughed. He continued to check things in there, then finished the examination. He asked me to get dressed and join him back in the other room when we were finished.

He told us that there was nothing physiological to be concerned about from my examination and then asked the simple question, "How often are you having sex?" We looked at each other, I replied that, "We don't keep count, but we make sure it's plenty around those days approaching and following what I think is ovulation anyway. Also, some in between, and it really varies from week to week."

He went on to talk about the fact that we all get too wrapped up in when we are carrying out the act. He said he feels that couples trying to get pregnant should do it every second day or more, and it shouldn't only be around ovulation, it should be all of the time to really ensure that you catch the egg after it has been released. Again, he mentioned the typical day 21 release, but said that this is not always the case for couples because people's cycle lengths vary. It can be earlier or later for some couples, so in order to make sure to catch the egg, you need to leave some fresh sperm in the tubes waiting for the egg. Don't make the egg wait for sperm; the sperm waits for the egg.

He explained that this sperm can live for 3-5 days, but the quality of the sperm depletes after a 24-hour period, especially if the conditions are in any way acidic in there. We then spoke about cervical mucus and its role. I could still never really tell the difference; I never knew if it was cloudy, or creamy, or sticky because, of course, it's all open to interpretation. If it is always thick and cloudy, then we may have an issue, but if you see some changes, it's probably fine. He advised me to drink lots of water to help this along.

I had spoken to a friend about her losses previously, and she mentioned that she had a procedure called a HyCoSy. This checks for any little issues in the fallopian tubes, such as blockages, and it's thought that having this procedure can often just dislodge anything that could be making it difficult for sperm to pass. She said that she got pregnant straight after it and swears by it. I mentioned this to the consultant, and he said, "By all means, I can organise that for you, but I don't think it's necessary." I told him I would think about that one and come back to him.

    He then spoke about progesterone, the hormone that helps maintain pregnancy, and said that my progesterone levels were slightly low according to the bloods, but nothing to be overly concerned about. He prescribed pessaries for whenever I might become pregnant. He seemed quite confident, to be honest, which was great. I had to use one of those in the morning and lie in bed for 30 minutes after insertion and then again in bed at night to help increase progesterone in the event that I did get pregnant. He then said he was going to send me downstairs to the pharmacy to get a hormone injection.

    After that, I was told to come back up and he would show me how to do it, so I could carry on doing it at home for myself. He told me that it is a form of HCG (Human Chorionic Gonadotropin), which is often given about 36 hours prior to egg retrieval for IVF. This helps to ensure that the egg or multiple eggs will be released in a predictable timeframe in the coming 24-36 hours to help to time intercourse, and to leave fresh sperm waiting for the egg.

    We went down to the pharmacy and got the injection. I was so excited; he seemed so positive and confident that this would be the answer. I was also nervous because let's face it, the prospect of injecting myself was not ideal. I'm not particularly afraid of needles or anything, but still, it's not nice to have to do it to yourself. All I can say is it's a good thing I was not relying on Mel to do it, as he is really not good with needles. We went back into the room. He took out the vial and needle and showed me the two separate needle heads and how to add the tablet to the liquid to complete the shot. He changed the needle head to the finer needle and showed me how to draw it up and get rid of the gas bubbles. He then pointed at the general area of the torso where I could inject and said to grab any loose fatty bits because it is not as sore to inject that way.

He pinched the skin and counted down, 3-2-1 and told me to do it slowly and gently, too, because you can damage the layers under the skin and get sore blister-like bubbles if you don't go deep enough into the tissue. I was relieved that it was done, and a sense of calm came over me. This could really be it; it's as simple as that. He gave me another 3-month supply of this injection to be taken on a particular day of my cycle by 12:00 in the afternoon.

He was very optimistic, claiming we didn't have any problems and we just needed to relax about it (which is the hardest thing to do). To go have fun and enjoy ourselves and not get caught up in the process, the woman's body is unbelievable, and it will do its own thing. He commented that stress is a real obstacle for pregnancy and told me to de-stress and stop worrying. I smiled and said, "Ok" (in my head thinking, "If someone could just actually tell me how because this is all I think about morning, noon, and night").

I asked him if it would be worth exploring things with my husband, and he said he didn't really think there was a need, but if I wanted to, we could. This part got to me for many reasons. Number one, it made me realise that I have been thinking all along that it's just me or something that I have done, that may have caused the miscarriage or the difficulty in conceiving. Number two, there seems to be such a stigma and a real sensitivity required when talking about the potential that the male may have some fertility issues, but this sensitivity is not given to women who are exploring their fertility health. It's always like a real insult to masculinity, should there be questions about male fertility, it's very taboo and embarrassing. Lastly, number three, why the hell should he not have his bits checked when I am being tested up and down and in and out, physically and mentally carrying the load of thinking that I am where the problem lies!!

The same consultant has a lab that carries out sperm testing, so we decided that we would bite the bullet and go ahead and get this done too, while the going is good. We were instructed to book that online when we got home.
I then asked about IUI and IVF, and whether we should pursue them if we still encountered difficulties in the future. The response of the doctor really set the tone for me about private healthcare. He replied, "I mean, I don't think you need to worry about any of those things if I am being honest, but this is private healthcare. If you want to keep spending money and you want me to do these things, I certainly can and will do them. You can call the shots here."

At this point, I had the feeling that he didn't have a vested interest in this process or in us per se; perhaps it was simply another opportunity for him? These comments made it feel like he was not in this for what I felt were the right reasons. We left it that I would get my results in 7-10 days, and in the meantime, we would book in for sperm sample testing. I had been given the HCG injection for that month, and I had three more to go. I had a prescription for progesterone, which I would start to use straight away if I get pregnant. The last words from him were, "I don't expect to see or hear from you again. I would be pretty confident that these shots will work. Now go home and get busy."

    We laughed and left with a pep in our step. We were so giddy and happy, so relieved to know there was evidently nothing wrong. We did a full analysis of the consultation on the way home, and we were really hopeful. I was relieved that we knew everything was ok on my behalf. The onus was not on me alone now. This was it; it was going to happen. Finally, some reassurance that everything was ok. Let's just ease off the pressure and have some fun again. This doctor knows what he is doing, he has seen it all. It's certainly going to happen within the next three months. He said so…clinging to every and any bit of hope and falsely promising myself it was going to happen. We tried not to be so regimental and just remembered the, "Every two to three days" rule for the entire month of August.

    The discussion began about the sperm sample. I knew it was something Mel probably wanted to avoid, but when I brought it to his attention again, he was more than happy to do his part. At least his part wasn't so invasive; he could do his bit alone and at least get some enjoyment in the process rather than having hands, heads, and utensils in his bits. But yet, it felt a little like his dignity had to be protected more than mine.

    We booked the appointment and then thought about the logistics. So, the booking email explained that a sample should be delivered no longer than one hour after ejaculation, but preferably forty minutes after. We wondered if they had rooms there you could use, like the ones you would see in the movies, but we learned that wasn't the case. We talked about what would be done to get the sample should a person get 'stage fright', but then again realised that we would need a room. I looked up hotels close by, but they were so expensive, and we just didn't have the cash that week, after paying a number of bills, and the honeymoon etc. Just normal life stuff, it was a tight week financially.

I knew this meant we would have to do a side-of-the-road job, but we certainly didn't need to be done for indecent exposure! I was afraid to openly say this to himself in case it would scare him off the idea altogether. But then, like that, I reminded myself that we all had to give up something here to make this happen, and then I didn't feel sorry for him anymore. After all, there were worse things you could be asked to do! Harsh...I know!

I opened Google Maps and inserted a radius of 45 km from the clinic. From there, we decided to find a quiet back road somewhere and try to get the job done, so to speak. It had to be close to the main road, of course, in order to get going and get the sample to the clinic before it would become defective for testing.

Sample day arrived. I felt like I had to tread carefully so as not to annoy or stress Mel out. The thought of doing this in the car in a public area was more than enough for a person to deal with. We packed up the car and headed off with all of the things we thought may be required, including sheets, etc to block the windows should stage fright kick in, and not forgetting a clean-up kit, just in case!

We smirked at each other a few times as we approached the general area that we knew fell within the travelling distance. I could feel the pressure building. I made a joke and asked, "So, have you chosen what you are going to watch for this now?" I thought I was hilarious, but Mel didn't quite agree.

We found a spot along the canal, just over a bridge and a little off the beaten track and said, "Ok, let's not dilly dally." We decided the best thing to do was that I would keep a lookout and leave him to it. We both felt anxious that someone would walk along the road or something. I thought it would take quite a while to do this on demand, but hey presto, to my surprise, the car door opened. The job was done within a few short minutes. I'm not going to lie; I was secretly proud of him for just getting the thing done.

Let's get a move on now and get this to the clinic. Well, I'm not joking with you, the comments and laughs were shocking on the way to the clinic. Such a relief, it was done. We could finally joke about it, but I did say, "Ok, I won't wreck your head about this anymore. That's it done now." Still, I can't help myself; we still have a laugh about it when the conversation ARISES!

I'm pretty sure so many other men and couples experience similar things. I spoke to one person I know about this, and she told me that her husband stopped at a well-known service station en route to the clinic, and went into the bathrooms there, and headed off up the road. There is nothing in place to facilitate men in this way for genuine purposes like this. To be fair, it leaves them in a STICKY situation...quite literally. I mean, what if someone CAME ACROSS them? They could be done for indecent exposure. Surely these clinics could have some provision in place within the centre to ensure viable samples. I know that in some clinics in the USA, they have rooms that you can use for privacy. I know I certainly can't imagine doing self-exploration in a public toilet or on the side of the road, so bravo to all of you men.

We got to the clinic, which was opposite the hospital, and I pulled up along the road. Off he headed, sample in hand. I was bursting to go to the bathroom, so I was delighted to see him walking back within a very short time frame. I asked what the person in the centre said, and he told me that he just took his details, the sample, and labelled everything and that the results would be emailed in a few days. I ran across to the hospital to go to the toilet and felt so happy. We were making progress, even if it was slow and brought us some news we didn't want to hear.

Again, I looked in awe at the big, round pregnant bellies in the hospital, and I remember thinking I really wish that was me, and hopefully it's going to happen very soon. We just had to persevere for what we really wanted. It always astounds me to think that for so many years I was the least maternal person you could meet, and now, I pined to be in that position, to be carrying my own baby, and to hold my own baby in my arms. I longed for that day.

Chapter Thirteen

The time to go back to school came along. It was now September 2022, and I was dreading it. I had to face people and try to carry out my job, but my mind was racing. I remember the drive to school on the first morning, and I bawled, crying the whole way in. I should be going back to school beaming from ear to ear, telling everyone my good news and showing off a little bump. Instead of that, I was miserable, desolate, empty, and traumatised. I was bursting to let this all out, but I had to hold tight for the shoulder surgery time off in just a few weeks; I couldn't start to let it out now, or there would be no going back.

    I remember driving with my head out the window, trying to calm my nerves and thinking I couldn't do this. I can't suppress this any longer. I parked the car a bit away, sat there for a few minutes, and pulled myself together. After giving myself a pep talk in the car, I got out and put on my fake smile and braved the day ahead. I remember the chit-chat before the first meeting, the usual questions like; "Oh, did you have a good summer?" "Did you do anything nice or exciting?" "Any news?" All innocent, and they usually wouldn't bother me, but I was trying so hard to hold myself together. I was almost ready to combust. I fought so hard with my emotions for those few weeks until I finally got to the Friday before my shoulder surgery.

The surgery was taking place on a Monday, and I said to Mel, "Ok. So, let's try to have a nice weekend because I need to let this thing entirely out after I get home from hospital."

I was a shadow of my old self. I hardly recognised myself anymore. I was so gloomy and my outlook on everything was bleak.

I had surgery on September 16th, and I got home the next day. The first two days at home were immensely painful. On the third day, I remember waking up and thinking, "Oh God, I can feel it. Today is the day I let this all pour out." I didn't know my arse from my elbow, I felt anxious and jittery, I felt panicky and found myself walking around the house aimlessly in circles, making massive jobs out of small tasks. I made some tea, sat down, and just cried. I started to think about where I could get help, and I began searching online. I read about psychologists and **counsellors** all over the country. I knew I was on the brink of unravelling, having kept all of this in for so long, so I needed help fast. I was happy to pay whatever I needed to get the help. I had to. I sent numerous emails and called many practices, all to no avail. The general message was that, if you call back in about 6-8 weeks, I might have freed up a space, but I have a waiting list. It was pointless. It felt like a dead end. This went on for days and days, and then one day, I was almost tipped over the edge.

In the meantime, I made myself get up, get showered, and dressed every day. I made myself try to do housework tasks and train Willo, play with the dogs, and rest loads to help with the surgery recovery. I was still tracking my period, mucus, ovulation, and taking the multivitamins that I was reading about, which would help with anxiety and restore balance.

September 27th came about, which was the next day that I had to give myself an injection. I set an alarm and woke up at about 6:00 am. Mel was already up, eating his breakfast. I went up to the kitchen to say good morning and got the injection from the fridge. I decided to go back to the room, lay everything out on the dressing table, and give myself a chance to wake up. I was going to be brave and just get it done and done right! I told Mel to leave the kitchen door open in case I needed him, but I wanted to do it alone and not be fussing. I took my arm from my sling and still had little or no movement in my arm. I washed my hands and sat down at the dressing table. I got the first needle head and I drew back the fluid and added it to the dissolvable powder. I changed the needle to the finer one and drew up the solution, ready to go. I held it up to tap out any air bubbles, and the liquid was far up the syringe, so I decided to **pull back the plunger a little more.**

    The next thing I knew, the part you drew back was in my hand, and the syringe was on the floor. The invaluable hormone liquid was on me and the floor. I froze for a minute, followed by a yell from the bottom of my lungs, screaming, "Noooooooo, no, no, no, no, no." Mel came running down; he had no idea what had happened. I was on my knees on the ground crying and saying, "I spilled it, I spilled it, Mel...I have ruined our chances again."

    I wasn't thinking straight. I panicked, and I was trying my best to draw it up off the floor into the needle again in sheer desperation. We only had two more attempts after this month with the prescription we had, and I literally just spilled our hopes for that month on the floor. This may sound irrational to some of you reading this, but in the state of mind that I was in, I lived in fight or flight mode, on the brink of a breakdown at any moment. This was heightened by anxiety and the fact that we had limited amounts of attempts with this apparent magic potion that was going to make it happen. The pressure to get it 'right' was unreal. It had to be timed perfectly. It had to be done before 12 noon that day. I was so mad at myself; I felt so stupid.

Poor Mel once again tried to comfort me, but I was in a state. I never felt so stupid and incompetent in all my life. How could I let a chance like that go? I was so stressed; I thought my heart was going to burst out through my chest. What the hell was I going to do now? It was too early to ring anyone, so I had to sit tight until 9:00 am. In the meantime, I calmed myself somewhat, but I had such jitters and a horrible feeling in my stomach. Mel eventually went to work. I knew I'd figure it out, but my mind was racing.

Time seemed to stand still, I had my fingers and nails eaten alive, I was in a sweat, I had clammy hands, and I couldn't focus on anything. I was like a hen on a hot egg! Thank God, 9:00 am came around. I decided to call my local pharmacy in Longford. I knew one of the owners, Siobhán in *Reilly's Totalhealth Pharmacy*, and she was really nice, I knew she would maintain confidentiality. This seemed like a big deal to me, that someone would know I was taking the shots at that time. They would think there was something wrong with me, and they would be watching me to see if they could figure out if I got pregnant after that or not. Again, an irrational, anxiety-ridden brain took over. I really don't know why this concerned me; look at the situation now, I have spilled every ounce of my previous insecurities into this book for everyone to see.

Either way, I called Siobhán and explained what happened through my blubbering voice and wobbling chin as

I spoke. Thank God I had been given back the prescription when I originally collected the shot from the hospital the day I was there. I sent her a picture of it, and she said to leave it with her and she would try to sort something out for me. I have to say, she was amazing; she was so understanding and showed great compassion. She didn't leave me waiting for too long, she understood the sense of urgency for timing and got to work on it straight away.

A short period of time passed by, and she called me back to say that she had called many pharmacies and nobody local had it in stock. It turns out that it was an unlicensed product, meaning it would only be available in pharmacies if ordered as a special item. I had gotten a dose the day I was in the hospital and brought one vial of the next dose home, and I was to pre-order the next one to be delivered to my local pharmacy when it was due, so I didn't have stock in the fridge. It's not something that they generally stock. She was going to try and call around a few more pharmacies in case someone had some that customers hadn't collected. She was so helpful and empathetic regarding the situation, and she really helped to calm me down. So, thank you, Siobhán. You helped more than you will ever know.

In the meantime, I was going to try to call the consultant's secretary. I tried and tried, but there was no answer. I emailed and got no reply. Siobhán called me back, but had no joy in her quest to call colleagues. A thought struck me, I had no other choice but to try the hospital pharmacy. Siobhán said she would call them to ask if they would send one down to her. In the meantime, I can ask the consultant's secretary to give me another prescription for the one I spilt.

The hospital told Siobhán that they could send it but it would be the following day at the earliest. That would not work; it had to be today before 12:00 noon, and it was now after 10 am. I said, "Ok, shoulder or no shoulder, I'll have to drive up." I asked Siobhán to tell them I would be up as soon as possible. Siobhán knew I had the surgery and **asked if I was sure I could go** and if should I be driving. It was only over a week since surgery. Thankfully, I had an automatic car, and it was my left shoulder, so I thought I would manage. To be honest, I didn't care. I was going to make this work. **I was determined to salvage a shitty mistake.**

I headed off as quickly and safely as I could. I won't lie, I was afraid I might be pulled over or something, so I took the sling off and hid it in case something happened, so I couldn't get into trouble. I was watching the minutes on the clock as we approached 12:00. The traffic was in my favour most of the time. I found a rare free parking space right outside the door. I didn't have time, nor did I care about paying for parking. I just had to get in there and get the shot, and after that, I didn't care. I was like a possessed woman. I hopped out, threw on the sling, and ran in as fast as I could. I wasn't even sure if I locked the car.

I went straight to the pharmacy and, thank God, there was nobody ahead of me. I explained the situation, and within 5 minutes, I had the shot in a bag. I didn't care about the shoulder now, it was 11:50 am, and I ran to the car. I opened the back door and jumped in. I pulled down the armrest and started to do the usual assembly. I paused, took a breath, and said to myself, "Laura, if you mess this up, you are absolutely stupid. Do it slow and do it right." I locked the car doors, and I remember whipping up my top, grabbing my belly, ready to go and saying to myself, "Right, no time to pussy-foot around. Let's go. 3-2-1 go." I stuck that needle in. I literally sighed, let a deep breath out, put the needle down, and rested my head back in the seat. I closed my eyes and rested there in a pure daze. I had been so wound up to this point that I could finally feel my heart begin to settle. Such a relief. I literally laughed and started thinking to myself, "Mother of God, if anyone saw me at this, they would think I was a pure junkie shooting up in the car." I needed a few minutes to gather myself again after what was an extremely stressful start to the day. We still had a chance now.

I drove home feeling more content and confident. I said to Mel, "If this works, it will make for a great story." A couple of days passed, and the dreaded two-week wait between ovulation and the wait to see if a positive pregnancy test would appear was dragging out. The old stress levels were heightening once again as the due date for my period approached.

Another period, another disappointment, and yet another kick to the face when I was already down. Utter devastation once again. After all of that effort!

Then came the most mentally challenging day that I think I've ever had. I'm not going into the details, but a typical disagreement between some family members in a WhatsApp group occurred, and some people shared some things they needed to get off their chest about me. That is fine because we all have those moments sometimes, and at least we get it out in the open and over and done with. We never stay mad for too long; we always get over it. Just a side note, we do all get on and I do love them.

Anyway, on this day, I was at my wits' end. I had spent the morning howling, crying, and frantically searching for someone to make my head feel better. I couldn't continue the way I was; I was an absolute wreck, completely inconsolable. I had spent a few minutes lying on the rug in the living room, where my legs went from under me, where I was crying so hard while Mel was at work. I felt weak both physically and emotionally. I was emotionally drained, and my energy was gone.

I started receiving messages in this group, and I just wasn't fit to get into a row or spend a day sending novels of messages to the group. I didn't have the energy, and my head couldn't focus. Then, another person in the group made their point as well. I did reply a few times and I said that, "I wasn't able for this conversation at the moment and I'll speak to you all soon. I'm just not in a good headspace and need space."

See, I hadn't really spoken to my family that much about this because it kind of felt like it was time I just got over it, even though nobody ever said that to me. Me, being me, I did what I always do. I try to do it all myself first, I am not good at asking for help, but it doesn't always feel like it's readily available either. Everyone is busy living their own lives too, as it should be. Everyone has their own life problems to deal with too, and I can openly say that I know I wasn't always there for them either. It's a two-way street, not a blame game. I put that down to the fact that I moved out of home at 18 years old and did my own thing.

I moved in with Mel and his mother about 15 minutes away from home, and I had more than one job at the time, and my own car shortly after that.

The conversation got heated, and a lot of things were said. I remember being on my knees on the floor with my head in my hands, tears rolling down my face, shouting at the phone as the messages were coming in, with me saying that I couldn't take any more of this, and if you only knew what was going on in my mind, you might fuck off and give me a break. I had literally told them that I was in a very low place, and still, the messages continued. That was so difficult for me, the one group of people who you should be able to turn to in a time of need had turned on me, even when I said I wasn't in a good place right now and couldn't cope at the moment. I was so overburdened with this heavy cloud, unable to shake it off. Everything was pressing down on me, and what would ordinarily be an argument resolved in a day or two became much bigger for me. During this period of vulnerability and uncontrollable thinking, this led to my first and only experience of truly suicidal thoughts, as I have mentioned earlier in this book. A very scary place to be.

At that very moment, I was completely out of control mentally – so deeply upset and at a loss – unable to see reason or to say, "Ah, fuck off" and put the phone away. I was unable to find the words to reply to the group to make it stop. I just thought to myself, "Well, if ever there was a time I would think about killing myself, this is it because I can't take any more, and at least my head would be at ease." It would all go away.

I wanted to text that in the group too, to make it go away, but then it felt like I couldn't, as it might seem I was merely looking for attention or an easy way out of the argument. I felt that I couldn't let them into my vulnerability. Nobody except Mel knew what was truly going on for me and how much I was struggling. I hid it quite well. One of the people from the group wanted to come to the house that evening and have it out face-to-face, but I just couldn't. I said no, let's leave it for a few days and let things cool off. We had visitors coming from the UK the next day for the weekend. I just needed to dust myself off and get on with that. Thankfully, that bought me a few days to try to pull myself out of the dark hole that I was in after being told that this was a prime example of what I do, that I always run away from my problems. Little did this person know I couldn't escape my problems, not even for a second. That was the problem.

  We met a few days later and sorted it out, as usual, it was just a heated exchange and a normal family argument- nothing out of the ordinary- but it felt like the straw that broke the camel's back at that time. I was still hurting at the fact that some of the people who are meant to have my back in a time of major emotional need couldn't put things aside and give me the chance I needed to sort myself out. It took me a while to move past that- I won't lie- but I had a bigger picture in mind, getting myself back to a reasonable and functioning state of mind. I just didn't want to argue, even still, I just want to live a happy, peaceful life with no drama. I can't be bothered giving it the energy that it consumes. Now I just don't get involved, and I deflect. It's just my mechanism for survival. This taught me to protect my peace and not let anyone else damage it or take it away from me. I don't love my family any less, this wasn't a terrible argument, I just couldn't handle it at that time. The main point is that in my unreasonable state, I couldn't take it. Usually, I would just say my part and move on.

  Do you believe in seeing or receiving signs? We received some signs from something/someone. I think these were signs to remind us that we should keep going, or that someone was watching over us to keep us safe, or sane, in my case. One thing worth mentioning is two visits from a white owl. One for me and <u>one</u> for Mel. You will probably read this and think I am making this up. But I really didn't. It's so strange because it only came at two intense times that were highly driven by emotion.

    A week prior to the UK visitors coming, Mel and I had an argument, it was only bickering. Nothing big or very important, but he didn't want to argue, so he just went outside and walked around the garden, so we could both cool off. He came back to the door and said to me, "Did you see it?" I replied, "See what?" (still cross, of course). He told me that he saw a white owl. I was thinking, oh right, yeah, ok...thinking he was half mad. We had a tree along the hedge dividing our site from a neighbour's farm, and one day they had a man in doing work in a digger. I saw an opportunity to have some of the hedge tidied up to give us an even better view of the area. I made the decision to do it while the digger was there clearing up the land, and that included taking the tree down (which has not been let go to date). There was literally one tree standing alone.

    Anyway, Mel was out walking around the tree to cool off. It was dusk, and he said the white owl swooped at him and flew around him quite low. He said its wingspan was massive, and it was hard to miss or mistake. It lingered around him, and even when he walked away from the tree back towards the house, it was still hovering around him. Then, he looked for it, and it was gone. Instantly, his gut told him it was a sign from his mother, like she was telling him to go back inside and sort things out. I remember we talked about it and I said, "I do recall your mother talking about that owl, but to be fair, I thought she was mistaking it for something else." She often told this story about a black rabbit living on the, lane, too and I never saw it, so I assumed it was that kind of a situation.

As I type this paragraph, a bird just flew right into the window...coincidence?

The visitors from the UK arrived. One of the nights that the visitors were here, I found myself getting upset. We were just sitting chatting and watching a film, and I was half reading a book. My mind was preoccupied by the dark cloud, but I was trying to put on a good show. I can't remember what the topic of conversation was, but I could feel the waterworks building up inside me. I said, "I'm taking the dogs outside for a few mins," so I could compose myself. I was pottering around the garden, throwing a ball for the dogs and trying to get some of the tears out quietly. All of a sudden, a loud noise caught my attention, it was the wings of a large white bird swooping by me quite close. I ducked and half-covered my eyes.

I stood up again and looked around. It was sitting in the tree, perched, staring at me. I couldn't believe it; it really was an owl. It was so big and looked so fluffy, almost like a cloud with eyes. It flew towards me again, but not as low, and circled over my head and flew off into the distance. I just stood in disbelief as it flew away into the darkening night sky. Straight away, I was thinking, "I wonder what this is a sign of?" I also felt like it was Mel's mother. I had a weird feeling in my gut, I felt shaking in my belly, like I felt nervous but also excited. I felt instant comfort and relief.

I was thirty-three when Mel's mother passed away. She was very much like another mother to me, as I lived with her for most of my adult life up to that point. Her passing really did impact me too, so I was happy to take this as a sign. We had never seen it before that, nor have we seen it since. I've been living in this area for approximately twenty years. I went inside, told Mel and the visitors, and I was all excited. I really felt a lift of positivity from it and took it as a sign to keep going. Everything would work out.

Chapter Fourteen

Now we are in October 2022 again. Every time Mel came home from work, he was greeted by a wound-up version of me, either standing at the door waiting for a hug, or he would find me crying as I explained I just need help, I need someone to help me, and I can't get help. God love him; he didn't really know what to do for me either. I told him about all the local community groups, family centres, private clinics etc. that I called each day so he could see how much I was really trying. I was in such a dark place. I was weak and vulnerable, and liable to potentially take some action to end it all.

And then it struck me, I remember speaking to a friend before who had lost more than one baby to miscarriage (she was based in a different hospital from the one I had attended). She told me about an on-site counsellor and how she was offered information leaflets, websites, and information on self care and the psychological care associated with this sort of loss. She egged me on to speak to the lady she had spoken to. In my sheer desperation, at my wits' end, I sent her an email explaining that I hadn't been a patient of that hospital, but her services were recommended.

I gave a brief synopsis of my situation and all the channels that I had used to try to get help, and asked if she could guide me in any way.

And there she was, my guardian angel! Within half an hour of sending the email, she replied, asking me if I lived far away. I told her where I lived. She said, "It doesn't matter what you are wearing or how you look, get into the car and come to see me and we will have a cup of tea and a chat." She gave me her mobile number and said to call her when I was outside, and she would come out to meet me. She was sympathetic and very willing to help.

Straight away, I felt like I could breathe fully again. I quickly threw on some clothes, hopped in the car, and headed off. I contacted Mel and told him that I think I have finally found a break. I think this woman might help me. Is it sad to say that I felt excited? I felt excited to think that I could possibly feel ok again. I felt like this might be the start of the end of the mental torture that I was enduring; it was really breaking me down bit by bit.

I got to the hospital and parked up, I rang her and she told me to wait inside the front door. I wasn't waiting long until she came along; I guessed that was her before she got as far as me. She just said, "Are you Laura?" I smiled and nervously said, "Yes." She smiled and said, "Come with me. We have a lovely space here for this kind of thing." As we walked along the corridor, she put me at ease as we chatted about general stuff. She took me to a family room that is there for use by people who have very sick babies or those who have received bad news about their precious baby. This was a very different setting compared to the one I had been exposed to in the other hospital I attended.

It wasn't long before I was reaching for the tissues as I spilled my guts to her about how things had been so difficult, I couldn't seem to move past this and that I needed help because I had been feeling so low. She listened and empathised with me, she validated how I felt, and she reassured me that this is normal, and that in time it will feel easier. The most important thing that she offered me was the acknowledgement of our little lost soul.

That's what I had been missing, acknowledgement and openness that this has happened and that it's ok for me to feel stuck!

Someone who acknowledged that this really does hurt, and it doesn't matter if it's a loss at 4 weeks or 40 weeks, that a loss is a loss and that we had so many plans made, imagined a life with this baby, and before we had a chance, it had been taken away from us. She told me that I should be able to talk about it and express my sadness without feeling like people don't care because it was so early into the pregnancy. She also reassured me that she encounters this a lot with women, and it's not just me. That is one of the reasons I decided to tell this very detailed story, to make others feel like they are not alone. Not the only one. She said that she often meets ladies who feel the same and feel shame.

It's typical that in modern Ireland we still can't talk openly about anything that might embarrass or upset someone, yet it's fine for them to be the first to keep asking, "Would you have kids?" and, "Why don't you have children yet?" and so on. Not only did this lady offer comfort, reassurance, and support, she also wanted to mark the existence of our little baby as a human. She told me that they hold a ceremony of remembrance every November for little babies who don't make it, and they offered to include ours in this ceremony.

I jumped at this opportunity.

I had to fill out a short form for the memory book. She then presented me with a little box with some bits in there including a journaling book, and information leaflets and to top it all off, she gave me a personal gift that was handmade by her mother. Her mother took up designing candles using custom jewellery as a hobby during Covid, and she wanted the counsellor, whom I will refer to as Lisa, to give one to families affected by loss so it could be lit every October for Baby Loss Awareness week in memory of their little loved and lost one(s). That candle sits by me on the desk as I write this, serving as a reminder.

Everything about this service felt so genuine and caring, it seemed like the first and only place that I was being truly understood, and not being made to feel like I just needed to stop talking about it and move on already! My vulnerability was being nurtured, it was allowed here, and I'm so glad I had found this place of comfort.

I sighed with relief during that first meeting. We ended it, and Lisa walked me the whole way out to the car and offered her help at any stage. I just had to send an email. I got into the car with all the bits she gave me, and I waited until she walked out of sight, I took a deep breath and smiled! A smile filled with relief and a sense of, "I'm going to be ok." I had finally been heard, and in the most genuine and frank way. It didn't feel false or forced, it felt just right. I drove home on a slight high, and I couldn't wait to tell Mel all about it and how I felt that there was a glimmer of light at the end of the tunnel. I was elated and felt lighter than I had done for some time. I could see the sense of relief on his face too.

Song: 'True Colours' by Mickey

This is a particularly beautiful version of this song. It's not a song I liked or listened to before. I remember sitting at the island in our kitchen, telling Mel about this sense of positivity at long last. He said, "I want to play a song that I have been listening to." So, it started, it was the song 'True Colours.' I never really listened to the words before, but they hit me hard. I knew he felt that they were about how he saw me at that time. He too was desperate to see my true colours come back!

    Mel didn't give up on me; he could see that the old me was still in there somewhere, and now the old me was trying to find the strength and way to come back! I realised that the words described us at that time. I cried; but this time it was with relief that I was still existing, that my soul was returning and that I could see that the world might be an ok place to be in again. Mel came and gave me a hug; it was like no other. We clung on to each other for a minute or so and didn't move. It was a special moment for us both that I will never forget. I knew he always loved and supported me, but this reassured me that he would always be there. Now, I knew I couldn't give up, and that there was some hope. It was a key moment that made us stronger than ever before. In a time of adversity, we became closer. We were all that we cared about now. Us, our health, and well-being. We had to prioritise ourselves over everyone else.

    Lisa offered to refer me to have counselling, and informed me that I was entitled to two sessions and recommended a lady practicing from home on behalf of the HSE. The first hospital I had attended certainly did not make me aware of any of this.

After a few days, I felt myself getting edgy again, waiting for this referral, and I emailed Lisa because I was really struggling. She was so comforting, reassuring, and supportive, and it didn't seem like any hassle to her to offer that open line of communication. I think she could tell I was desperate, so she contacted the counsellor again and then the process sped up. The lady had been on leave, but Lisa told me to come and see her again to offload while I waited for the appointment. That I did.

It felt that no matter who we spoke to or where we went, the conversation turned to people expecting babies or chatting about babies, and this was killing us. I guess we were hypersensitive to this topic now.

For some reason that year, October was really highlighted as the month when you light a candle in your window on a certain date to remember lost babies. God bless the algorithms. I had the handmade candle from Lisa's mother and I decided to light it in front of the telly. I felt embarrassed to put it in the window in case anyone would think I was milking it or looking for attention. Can I add, we live up a Cul De Sac lane, it was not likely anyone would see it. I still don't understand the shame. I also noticed loads of people posting on social media with pictures of their candles lit and little rainbows or angels after their post. I learned that the number of rainbows or angels represented the number of losses people had. Firstly, I was taken aback by the number of people I knew who had losses. Some had multiple. I can't express enough sympathy to you if that is you. I sat and stared at the flickering flame while we relaxed, watching telly that night. I remember having to blow it out before bed, and it felt like I was saying goodbye and letting go all over again.

Moving on from that, a relaxing Saturday morning came about. Mel got both of us a coffee, and we stayed in bed for a while and relaxed. Then it was time for another injection. As I already mentioned, I was generally grand with needles, but I really wasn't excited about doing it to myself. I had no hesitation with the previous shot because I was under severe pressure. I felt edgy about this one, given the experience of the last one. I gave myself a pep talk and said, "Just do it." It wasn't painful when the consultant did it. I didn't even feel it last time in the panic that I was in. Get it done and shut up. I washed my hands, followed the instructions exactly, and even watched a YouTube tutorial just to be sure. I took the vial, which had a dissolvable tablet in it, and left it on the bedside locker. I took the syringe and the larger needle head and pierced the foil on the liquid solution. I drew up the liquid solution as per instructions and then pierced the foil on the dissolvable tablet, I pierced it and squirted the liquid in to dissolve the tablet. That was it. That was the magical solution.

    I changed the needle head to the smaller, finer one. I pierced the foil again and drew up this magical potion, making sure to get every last drop. It was time to lie down and pinch the gut to get a good fatty bit, reducing the chance of feeling the injection. I had clammy hands, and I felt nervous. I said to myself, "Ok, let's go," but my hands didn't move...I laughed nervously. I took a breath and said, "Ok, this time, now I'll do it." I counted down 3...2...1...go, and I paused. I didn't move again. The hesitation made me feel even more nervous and mad at myself for being such a chicken. I was willing to do anything at this stage for a baby, but I was finding this so difficult. I thought to myself about all the women out there who had done this dozens of times, and some who have done it hundreds of times, and I thought to myself, "You are such a pussy. Just do it, it will be over in a second, so just MAN UP!"

Again, I lined things up, I got a pep talk from Mel, and he counted down this time. 3...2...1...go...I moved my hand with the needle to my skin and stuck the very tip in, and I panicked...I removed it, and I got mad. Mel offered to do it for me. Now, as I mentioned earlier, he is an absolute wuss with needles. If he saw me having a cannula in my arm, he would have to look away and would almost be sick, so the thoughts of him doing it was totally laughable.

He said, "I'm not going to do it gently though; I'm just sticking it in." I replied, "Eh no, the doctor said to do it gently or it will be very sore and to release the fluid steadily and slowly." After that, I decided that I was not going to let him do it. I was ready, at long last. Ok, 3...2...1...go, and I finally did it. I stuck it in slowly, and then I kind of froze with it in there and started to breathe heavily. I slowly moved my hand into position and released the fluid. I did it, and it was stinging. I obviously didn't go deep enough, because it caused a bubble to appear at the top of the skin. When I saw that, I was furious with myself yet again.

For God's sake, I made such a song and a dance about that, and I fucked that up too. Great, I convinced myself that I couldn't get pregnant this month either because I didn't inject deep enough. A rollercoaster of emotions followed. Firstly, I was relieved and proud that I had done it. The shakes and cold clammy sweat finally disappeared. Secondly, I was raging with myself for not doing it right and the blame game kicked in again as I trawled through my thoughts, annoyed with myself. After yet another hissy fit, full of tears and irrational blame, I pulled myself together and got on with the day. I tell you all of this in such detail because I want to highlight the fact that I became so hard on myself. In my eyes, everything I did was wrong or not good enough, and I felt like a failure. It is a terrible cycle of blame and guilt. That's the thing about this entire process; not a day passes where you don't blame yourself. I never once automatically blamed Mel in all of this. I assumed it was all on me, all my fault, and that I was doing something wrong all the time.

  A new week started again. Why is none of this easy? It is obstacle after obstacle...and then, Occupational Health started ringing me to see if I'm fit to return to work after my surgery. I probably was physically fit, but mentally, I was nowhere near ready to face the world. Due to this, I had to make sure that I could remain off work, but as it turned out, they wanted me to take an extra five weeks on top of the recommended six weeks (based on the type of shoulder surgery).

  I couldn't afford to use my full-pay sick leave, so I pushed to go back after the planned six-week mark as recommended by the doctor. This was just another thing to worry about; would I be forced to go back earlier than I was fit to or indeed stay off longer than I could afford to? I didn't want to tell them about the state of my mental health because I was afraid it might have consequences. Don't ask me what the consequences were, but I felt like I couldn't mention it. It was a totally separate issue.

  Eventually, I got an appointment for counselling and I went to the counsellor's house. It was unusual as it was located on a farm, yet it was a HSE service, but it felt homely. It was nice because I literally felt like I was in someone's sitting room. She welcomed me in and was very nice, and we chatted before getting down to business. She asked me why I was there, sincerely acknowledging the loss and my feelings. Mind you, the message that I probably gave across at the time was the feeling of a lack of support and help, and the feeling of being isolated in dealing with this. We ended up going off on a tangent, which I don't deny was probably needed. But in my mind, it wasn't addressing what I felt needed to be discussed at this point. The focus ended up being on something totally different from a comment I made in passing.

I sat through the session and we talked a lot, but I noticed the therapist watching the time, and by God, on the dot of the hour, that was that. It was the end of the session. We were going away to celebrate our first wedding anniversary that night, so I told her I would contact her in a week or so to make the next appointment. I never did, though. I didn't feel that she was right for me.

I didn't have a connection, and I felt it was a waste of time as it wasn't addressing what I needed at that time.

I think that you really need to find someone that you can connect with, someone who is really listening to what you are saying and what you want to talk about, and not redirecting the conversation. Again, I say she was very nice, but just not for me. I got into the car and I called Mel, telling him it was grand but I wouldn't be going back. It just didn't feel right, and I couldn't wait to get home and head away for the night with my wonderful husband.

On the drive to the hotel, I told Mel about the counselling session, and then I said, "Ok, let's not talk about it this evening, or for the rest of the night. We need a break." At that, we encountered a double rainbow.

We both smiled and felt that it was a sign. I thought I was going to be ok, and the baby is looking down on us.

We had a fantastic time, drinking lots and talking into the small hours. It's like the hotel was celebrating our anniversary too; they kept giving us free prosecco, cocktails, and a few little shots. We hadn't been drinking much in the last while, as we were trying for a baby, and my mood was low, so this break was exactly what we needed. I also knew there was no chance I was pregnant because I had my period, of course, it is always guaranteed to align with social events and plans! The consultant said to us that he obviously doesn't recommend drinking regularly or binge drinking, but a few glasses of wine can help to calm the situation when you need to relax and take your mind off things. That wasn't an invitation to go get 'smashed' mind you.

The arrival of this period also meant that we didn't conceive following the hormone injection. This was devastating. I had myself convinced that this was all it was going to take. After all, the consultant said that the timing and conditions at the time of the shot that he administered were perfect. Everything was lined up, so he didn't even think that I would need to use any further shots. In my head, that was it, I was sure I would be pregnant. It was like getting a slap in the face, if I am being honest. I had to become numb to it because I just couldn't accept it. Medically, everything was aligned for it to happen, and it hadn't. We had one shot left for November.

We were having a great night in the hotel, dinner was lovely, the bar was hopping, and drinks were flowing. We headed back to the room after some time wandering around the castle. When we got there, I let my guard down. The reality of this shot not working had been lurking and trying to take over; add the drink-infused mood to that, and it was a recipe for a disaster. Such anger and upset ensued. We had a talk; well, I had a cry and gave out, and poor Mel just listened to me once again as I wailed and exclaimed how unfair all of this was. Then, of course, the guilt kicked in; I blamed myself for ruining our first anniversary and taking from what was a really enjoyable night. There was no combatting these bastarding feelings; it was impossible. What was meant to be a nice, relaxing night away, restful and reviving, turned into a massive hangover, lower mood than before, swollen eyes from crying, and guilt for ruining the night. Why could I not just hold things together and park it all in the back of my head?

    Monday morning came, and we were back to reality. The next thing was that ovulation was looming again, which meant that it was soon time to inject again. According to my app and my calculations, I was due to inject Saturday morning before 12:00. The usual craic was going on in the background for the full cycle, counting days on the app, tracking the start and finish date of my period, and noting the flow. Noting the mucus and changes, trying to feel for the opening of the cervix, peeing on ovulation sticks, and Googling the instructions multiple times to read them and ensure I was not missing something. The same exhausting level of obsession, consumption, and self-torture!

    It was time to follow up on test results for me (bloods) and Mel's (sperm). Such a job to get them. My goodness, for a private service, it was harder than trying to drain blood from a turnip, considering that a few hundred euros had been exchanged already for the pleasure of these tests.

    I called the secretary several times and emailed frequently to try to get the results. After numerous messages on the answering machine and efforts to contact her, I gave up for a week. Eventually, the following week, I got her on the phone and she told me that she would speak to the doctor and call me back. She didn't call me back, so after a few days, I decided to call her again. I was furious. She had no idea of the mental drain this was already having, without chasing her to do her job. The same saga went on and on, and eventually I got her again. She told me that she would email them to me. I was delighted, that's great, I thought to myself.

Then, of course, the email never came. So, the saga continued of calling and leaving messages, and being left wondering if there was something wrong or what. Then one day, I received an email with an attachment only and no explanation. It was the sperm sample results with loads of medical terms, percentages, and results. I had no idea what was what.

There I go again to Dr. Google, searching all of the terms on the sheet and searching for the result ranges to see where we were on them. It was mind-boggling. I couldn't quite figure out if it was in the normal range or if it was abnormal. I emailed back, thanking her for the results, and inquired whether it was normal or if we needed to do anything further. Another week passed by, and she informed me that if I wanted to speak about the results, I would need to pay another €250 for an online consultation. All I could do was say, "Yes, let's organise it." Then, she told me the doctor wouldn't be available until the following week. I made an appointment and got off the phone. I went into overdrive again. All I could think about was, "Oh God; there is something wrong if he wants to talk to us about the results." It was nerve-racking.

The call with the doctor took approximately two minutes for him to basically say that, everything is perfect in the sample, and we have nothing to worry about (thanks for the money!). Goodbye. All that wasted time worrying unnecessarily, which added to the stress that he told me I needed to reduce in my life. Instead, he was the cause of it, throughout that waiting period, and all for nothing. It was just more money spent when they could have replied, "Yes, this falls in line with the expected results", or "No, we would like to discuss this further with you and your partner."

Anyway, we were relieved all the same.

Chapter Fifteen

Ok, so what is next? November 2022 was soon coming around, which meant we had one last injection to go. At this stage, I was really contemplating IUI, basically artificial insemination of sorts. I was looking up the cost and where to get it done. I wasn't even considering the consultant from before.

It was at this moment that I remembered the idea of having the HyCoSy test done. The way it was described to me, in simple terms, was that it's a test to look at your tubes and internal reproductive bits, and to see if there is any sign of endometriosis or other issues going on in there that might delay or prevent conception. I spoke to a woman who had this procedure, and she swears that it is what helped her with her pregnancy. Apparently, it can dislodge any potential blockages that might be making it difficult to conceive. I decided to go to my GP and ask for a referral. What was there to lose?

I received an appointment for later in November. I was delighted because it would fall just before ovulation, so in my mind, I was sure that this would clear the way for any blockages, identify if there were any issues, and it would be done on time for the last of my injections. This was certainly going to be a winner; I had all avenues covered for this cycle. It is amazing how you spend so much of your time calculating and planning, all in the hope that it will work out. You don't hesitate, but you will try anything in desperation.

I had been reading about the procedure and what it entailed. I read real women's stories on 'Mumsnet' and another fertility support group on Facebook called 'Don't tell me to relax!' The name of this was very appropriate, all the professionals advised me to just relax...just relax and it will be fine.

It was an internal scan, and while they were in there, they would insert a tube with a balloon attached. They inflate the balloon, and a fluid is added to detect any blockages or scar tissue in there. It is as if the inflating balloon helps to widen the tubes and leave a clear passage for the sperm.

Might I add that reading about this stuff is very complicated. I noticed what seemed to be like a second language or a code with abbreviations for medical terms and other related terms. It took me so long to figure these out, so here are a few to help you along if this is new for you;

TTC – Trying To Conceive.

2WW – Two Week Wait between ovulation and your period (this seems to take an eternity when you are hoping for that positive test).

FSH – Follicle Stimulation Hormone blood tests check for the follicles on the ovary and their growth to prepare eggs for ovulation.

HCG – Human Chorionic Gonadotropin is a chemical that is usually present in early embryos and the levels of this hormone can indicate if a pregnancy is occurring, or if a pregnancy is being, or has been lost.

BBT – Basal Body Temperature is where you use a thermometer the moment you wake up and chart the change in temperature each day. This indicates a slight change in body temperature prior to ovulation, alerting you to the fact that it's time for business.

LH Sticks – **Luteinising** Sticks or ovulation strip tests. You pee on these, and the strip indicates whether the luteinising hormone is present or not. This indicates whether it is a good time for business or not.

DC – Darling Child.

DH – Dear Husband.

DD (1) – Dear Daughter (1st one). The number indicates the order of the children, not the age.

DS (1) – Dear Son (1st one). The number indicates the order of the children, not the age.

This is my understanding, anyway. But be sure to consult a qualified medical professional!

It was the day of the HyCoSy test in November. I had read about some people's uncomfortable experiences, but I had convinced myself that I would be grand and that I am ok with some amount of pain. I also told myself that those people are probably just being dramatic; I didn't mean that as an insult to them, but rather as a coping mechanism for myself. I was telling myself it would be ok.

Mel and I headed up to a different hospital for the test. I was not looking forward to the process; however, I was giddy at the prospect that this could be the missing piece of our puzzle. It made sense. Clear any blockages, inject the hormones, and get that sperm in there. It couldn't be easier...right?

As we approached Dublin, there was a traffic jam due to an accident. We had allowed loads of time because the appointment wasn't until 11 am. We were hoping to miss all of the morning traffic. We were 15 minutes from the hospital but had 50 minutes to spare. Time moved on, but the traffic jam caused by the accident did not. I was panicking. I didn't know what to do. Would we make it, would we not? Then, of course, all I could think about was that my perfectly calculated plan wouldn't work because I would have to reschedule again, and I wouldn't have any more injections, and my mind went into a negative spiral. In fact, I don't think there was a day that this sort of thing didn't happen. I lived in fight or flight mode each and every day.

    It was 10:50 am, and all I could think of doing was calling the hospital. The traffic was starting to move, but very, very slowly. I was really upset, thinking that I wouldn't be accepted any later than my appointment time. Thankfully, I spoke to someone who was extremely nice. She told me to come ahead and not to panic that they would leave me to the end and see me then. This was such a relief. The pressure was off a little.

    We finally got there at about 11:25 am. I ran to the area and checked in after getting lost in the wrong building first. I was taken to a small changing room and given the obligatory sexy blue gown. I waited and waited, and I was afraid I was forgotten, so I opened the door. It was on a very busy corridor and I certainly did not need to flash my bits at any passers-by, so I ensured all the bits were in. I was really nervous. Mel had gone to park the car and then followed me in, but it was all such a rush, I didn't get to tell him where I was for ages. I told him it's hard to find the place, and I shouldn't be too long. I told him to wait at the main reception area, have a coffee, and I'll come find him afterwards. It was hard for him to be back in that hospital environment. Only a very short time before this, his mother had been a patient there, and she underwent treatment and surgery. She passed away in September 2019. It was a horrendously difficult period, so all of that came flooding back for him.

I was called into the room. There was a large bed with foot stirrups (I was getting used to these now, and not for any fun reason). There was an internal scanner, a few storage presses, a metal trolley with tubes containing all sorts of things, and a sheet to cover my dignity for a few minutes. I was chatting to a lovely nurse who put me at ease. She said the doctor will be in soon.

He came in, and the atmosphere shifted from a bubbly, warm, gentle tone to an efficient, formal, and more serious atmosphere. He was very cordial, mind you, and explained everything to me in detail, but he was all business. He asked me to scoot down to the bottom of the table and bend my legs up. He then asked permission to begin the exam. He used a condom on the magic wand on the scanner with a small helping of lubricant and slowly began his work. It was nothing more than slightly uncomfortable for the first few minutes as he moved around and had a good look at all the bits and bobs in there. Then he said, "Ok, let's prepare to inflate the balloon." This is the part I had been reading about, but I was ready. I braced myself. I was also telling myself, "Don't clench, don't be tense, let things be loose, and it won't be as painful."

The inflation started, and as it inflated, the pain got sharper and sharper. Not totally unbearable by any means, but I definitely knew that things were being stretched to their absolute limit. It felt like an internal 'Chinese burn' paired with severe period cramps.

He released the fluid into the area and used the magic wand to check for anything beyond the norm. He then had to do it on the far side. I was sweating and dreading it. He started it again, on the far side, and this time I knew better what to expect, but I found it worse. He was talking away to the staff about what he was observing. There was also a trainee doctor in the room, as well as a floating nurse who was coming in and out as the test progressed, opening and closing the door out to the busy corridor with my bits exposed and facing the door. I was a bit anxious about that door opening and closing, but at that stage, anyone could have their head up there, to be honest. I was in pain now, trying to stay still. I had closed my fists, grasping onto the sheet. My palms were clammy; I felt a tear running down my cheek. I was exhaling very loudly, trying to control my breathing, but it was so hard.

He inserted the fluid and continued to examine things. He reassured me that I was doing very well and we were almost done, to hold tight, and keep breathing. The nurse came to me and asked if I was ok, she then asked if I felt dizzy. She said that women often faint because they forget to breathe, so to take deep breaths.

She did some breathing with me, and this really helped to calm me down a little and relax my body which, in turn, made the examination a little easier and quicker. The doctor then said, "Ok, let's deflate the balloon," and warned me that there would be lots of fluid when he does that, so not to worry if I feel fluid coming out. As he deflated the balloon, I had a very intense pain, a pain like I had never experienced before. It's so hard to describe. I was doubled over the end of the bed and couldn't talk. The doctor asked me if I was ok, and I knew I was. I knew that it would pass, but it still really hurt.

He removed all the tubing and everything else that was in there, and I relaxed my legs and body. I was so relieved; in my head, I was saying, "Oh, thank fuck for that." I lay with my eyes closed for a moment and continued to breathe hard, still holding my stomach.

He explained that the test came back clear, that everything was in full working order. He had no issues or concerns with anything that he saw in there. He said there was a partial blockage on one side, which they cleared out with the balloon, but it wouldn't have caused any issues. He instructed me to sit at the end of the bed, take my time to get dressed, and then leave the room, and a report would follow to my GP. He then left the room, and the nurse took over with kindness.

I was still lying flat with a small sense of shock, to be honest. They left me there for a few minutes to gather myself. Then the nurse asked me if I would like some water. She offered me a hand to sit up, but told me not to rush, as I could get dizzy. After, she gave me some pads and paper towels. She told me where to leave the paper towels when I had finished, and she left the room once she knew I was ok. At this point, I was glad that the secretary who called me to give me the appointment told me to take two Ponstan (pain relief) prior to arriving. I didn't have any because I don't like taking medicine, so I took paracetamol. That just didn't cut it here!

Once the nurse left, I squatted down to the ground and curled up in a fetal position with the pain. I paused there for a few minutes and I reminded myself that this was all for a good cause, and I was glad to have had it done. I slowly made my way to where I had left my phone and texted Mel, saying that, "I would be there soon." I looked back at the bed and noticed quite a bit of blood, given how I felt, I wasn't at all surprised. I felt bruised and tender, but slowly it was easing. It wasn't taking my breath away anymore. I stood up and tried to walk to my clothes, but I had to move slowly. I just wanted to get out to Mel, so I got dressed quickly and left the room. I was walking so slowly as I still had strong pains, certainly enough to barely walk along. I could see Mel in the distance, and I started to get emotional (again, I know!) I couldn't wait for a hug. He saw me coming and came towards me with a face of concern and worry, and gave me a hug. I needed to sit down, so we found a seat and I told him all about it. He went and got me a coffee and some cake to make me feel better, of course. Cake always helps! I had to get the blood sugar back up, you know!

    I was still feeling some pains, but now they were much more bearable. I still couldn't attempt to walk to the car park yet. I did get up to go to the toilet and felt a gush of fluid. I was afraid to look, to be honest, but the pad they had given me had done the job. I took my time in the bathroom and came back out. I needed five more minutes before the walk back to the car. I was smiling again. Glad it was over and still glad I got it done. Would I do it again? Absolutely, yes! At that stage, if I had to jump into a fire to be told that I would have a baby, I wouldn't have even contemplated it, I would have done it straight away. I finished the cake; I couldn't leave any of that behind! Then we headed back to the car hand-in-hand, glad that another step had been taken towards us having a baby.

    We were really also reassured that there was nothing sinister or obvious showing in the examination. This gave us a boost, and it was a positive way to head towards ovulation and the last injection. So, I had clear tubes, was more tuned in to recognising my signs of ovulation, and I had this hormone injection to take. Without a doubt, this was going to be the month.

In the midst of all of the emotions, appointments, and disappointments, I started to feel a flicker of faith. This is an odd one for me. I spent years saying, "I don't believe in anything. Sure, when you are buried, you are buried, and forgotten in no time." I was very much in the mindset of thinking it's all pure imagination. To be honest, I have often said before that if a man today claimed all the things that Jesus apparently did, that they would be in a straitjacket before long. Something changed, though. For me, it's not about the wondrous stories or the make-believe characters in question, nor the prayers and believing that the prayers will fix everything. It's about allowing yourself to have a space to deload and have free thoughts to the person or people that you miss. I think I had gotten to a point where I had nothing else to cling on to apart from hope, and I was willing to do whatever I needed to remain positive.

When I met Lisa, she told me about a ceremony of remembrance that they carried out every November in the Cathedral in that town. This ceremony was to acknowledge and remember all of the losses recorded in that county for that year and previous years. Any family that has been impacted by fertility/maternal loss or that is grieving the loss of a young person was made to feel welcome. I had taken the form home to fill out because I knew I needed to be in the right headspace to do so, and I wanted to include Mel in that part. There were the usual questions, such as age of gestation, gender, and a section for the name. This brought a new wave of emotion, as I felt like I didn't even get a chance to get to know who was in there, to give them a name.

Who did I lose? How can I say goodbye when I don't know who you are, little one?

I found that quite challenging, but of course, it was far too early to know that, so I just put the name as 'baby Doyle'. The illogical, intrusive thinking kicked in again. It made me feel like I had no right to grieve, that I was being completely foolish for doing so. After all, I didn't even know this little being. Then pair that with the comments such as, "Ah, it could be worse, imagine being further on," and the like. This made me feel even more foolish for feeling what I felt. Like I had nothing to be complaining about, and that I couldn't talk about it. It made me feel embarrassed. Embarrassed that I was in such upheaval over something that everyone had suggested didn't really matter. They did this with either thoughtless comments or by pretending to listen and care, but their facial expressions, bored eyes, or body language didn't convey genuine care or attention to the matter. It felt like I was being plámásed just so people wouldn't feel bad. I got the feeling from a few people that they were awarding me the grace of asking, but didn't really show interest of truly caring about the impacts. This was simply because they didn't get it, or that they were too selfish to see beyond themselves for a moment.

In turn, I felt angry at myself for allowing myself to feel embarrassed. I was mad at myself for not telling people they had no clue and to shut up when they made those flippant comments.

Sorry. That was a side rant. Now back to faith and the ceremony of remembrance.

We didn't know what to expect, so we headed off and went into the cathedral and took a seat. There was a massive crowd, which I had not anticipated. I found myself gazing around at people and families, wondering what their story was like. Some of them had other children, and I wondered what that was like. Were they truly happy again with their families, or do you ever feel better again? I was half afraid to look around in the event that I knew other people there who didn't know our story.

I noticed that many people there had supportive families of siblings, parents and grandparents along with them. I'm not going to lie; I know I was a little envious of that. They were part of the healing process, something neither of us felt that we had. I had mentioned the ceremony to some family members. To be fair, we didn't tell everyone, but we did share it with a few. It almost felt embarrassing that we would consider doing such a thing. Almost like we were being dramatic about the whole thing, but we weren't, we were devastated, broken and absolutely saddened. When we said that it was coming up, we were met with quietness and, in some cases, blank facial expressions that told us that they didn't really think that it was necessary, so then we just didn't tell anyone else about it.

There was a magnificent display as we entered. There was a tree up near the altar, with each leaf representing a loss to some family, and my goodness, those leaves were plentiful. They were cut out on coloured paper and individually hung. There were loads of other beautiful representations along the way, and most of the participants in the ceremony were young children themselves — siblings of those who had been lost. It was so lovely to see them as happy as could be, representing their loved one and bringing so much joy to the cathedral.

There were some poems, songs, and some artwork by children, and much more. It was very personal and inviting.

We felt that our baby was finally acknowledged just the same as everyone else's that day, without question or judgement. Just as it should have been from the start. There was a unique sense of collective support there that day as everyone had a different story or experience, but everyone had the same outcome, a loss. Here, it was ok to make a little fuss over them. We were finally allowed, and it was fully accepted in this place. A place of connection and solitude at last.

There were tears, but also a new sense of warmth that day. It felt that somehow, in this place, the cathedral, we had a connection to this little person who should have been, and we were in no hurry to leave at the end. From this day, I started to light candles in there. I wasn't saying prayers to God or Mary or the usual suspects. I was lighting a candle and having a small word in my head with that lost soul. It felt that there was a presence in this place.

Again, I think a lot of this comes down to hope. Hope they can hear your thoughts, telling them how much you love and will miss them, and how much you wish you had got to know them better. Hope that they can hear you pleading for help, to clear your head, and to help you to become more positive. Hope that they can hear you thinking about all the images in your head of what being a mammy to them would have been like. Hope they can hear you thinking about the fun and love that they would have experienced with you, so that they can rest easy too and know that they were deeply loved. I asked why it had to happen, and of course, I didn't get an answer. Who knows?

I was never religious, and I don't think I am now either; however, certainly, faith in something has been ignited in me. I never thought about faith like this before, but now it felt like it was different. It had to be different if I was going to make it through and be ok. Mel and I agree that when you are there, it feels like you are really communicating and being heard by those people that you want to connect with in your thoughts.

I had a ritual; I would light a candle for Mel's mam, and I always had a few things to say to her. Then I would light a candle for Mel's dad, whom I never met, but I always said a few things to him, and then I would light a candle for the baby. For a moment, it felt as though they could hear me. In fact, we were sure that we were getting signs. Maybe it's coincidence, maybe it's our brains in a sense of false hope of connection to the baby. Either way, does it really matter once it brings comfort and solace to you? Even if it is a placebo effect. We still go to churches regularly to light a candle and have a sit and think.

There were loads of small things like white feathers in unlikely places, far away from doors and windows, and then, the white owl. There were times when we needed money, and we asked these people to give a handout, and money always came along. There were loads of things.

I remember a conversation with Mel's mam years ago. She had great faith, and I never understood why, because she had a lot of sorrow after losing her husband young. I asked, "Why do you bother going to Mass? Do you believe that you will go to heaven, or what is it?" She said, "If you don't have faith, you don't have hope, and if you don't have hope, you have nothing!" Maybe that was it; maybe I felt there was hope that our little baby would hear us and likewise, that we would feel like we were heard by loved ones.

Now I understand that maybe she felt that same connection with her lost husband. I never understood it that way. I used to think that when you had some sort of belief and went to mass regularly that it was a form of brainwashing, to believe in stories of characters. However, now it's something totally different to me, and I think I finally understand why people go. Everyone has their own experience or view of it, but this is what it now means to me.

Speaking of loss, I want to address the loss of Mel's parents. This has been hugely significant to both Mel and me. I started going out with Mel a year after his dad passed away unexpectedly in their home. I never got to meet him. His name was Sean. I heard so many fond stories and memories of him. I always wondered if he would have liked me or merely tolerated me, but I like to think it would be the former. He was very caring and loving to his wife and family, well thought of in the local community, and a real messer at heart, so I believe. I was so young when we got together.

I had never really encountered such grief from anyone up until this stage of my life. I had encountered grief and loss, yes, but I had never seen a family more scarred from the same. I must have been coming and going to the family home for at least two years before I could directly ask what happened, and even then, words were limited to just a few. They just found it really hard to adjust to it and accept it. Who wouldn't? Mel faced his own battles with this for years, and he had some very dark times. He always thanks me for sticking around for him because who knows where he would be or what he may have done…He tells me that I saved him. As a young person, it was hard to help him; all I could do was be supportive and loving.

The year after this, two of Mel's best friends died tragically in a car accident. Another blow to a young man who was already hurting. It was very hard to deal with this. I was so young I didn't know how to handle it properly, but I did my best.

Then, in 2019, Mel's mother passed away. Her name was Mary Rose. We had just started building our home. She never got to see it finished nor join us on our wedding day. She spoiled him rotten in her own little way. I used to slag him about being a mammy's boy! He got away with murder because he was her youngest and, in her words, "My Mel." Even in his 30s!!!

I also had developed a very close relationship with her as she really did become a mother figure to me. We used to knock heads occasionally, never anything major, but we would always have a laugh fighting over the first slice of her renowned fresh treacle bread. God love her, we would come in drunk after a night out and lie on top of her in the bed for the chats. Mel would make her give him a hug, and she would shout, "Go away, you stink!" She secretly loved it…as did we. She pretended she didn't care, but she often brought us tea and toast in bed the next day to help us come back to life.

The loss of his parents became so important along our journey. The level of support would have been so different, whether it was wanted or not. Mary Rose would have been there to, "Check if the post came," or to "Peel a few spuds," or something like that, just to get a chance to check in on us. We never spoke about emotional stuff, but that was the emotional support right there. That, or a bowl of semolina or tapioca with extra sugar.

Mel was explaining to me recently that, as a man, he feels that looking back, he did need to speak to someone about the loss of our baby and the whole experience. Also, he felt that he didn't have someone close enough to talk about it with, without feeling embarrassed or less manly (God forbid). He did speak to one person, but he didn't get into it too much because that's not what you are meant to do as a man in traditional Ireland!

His mam and dad would have been that support for him. He always says that one big regret that he has is that he was twenty years old when his dad died, and never really got to have a chat with his dad to get advice from someone who was doing such a great job at parenting. It never entered his thoughts at that stage. He was enjoying life—going out with friends, doing his own thing—but he never got to go for pints with his dad or have those long, deep conversations with the one person he could have truly confided in. He feels that he missed out on having those lines of communication by not having a parent to turn to.

He jested and mentioned the secret man-code, which is, of course, where you don't talk about those emotional things. He told me that he can't remember any of his male counterparts or uncles ever crying or really getting very sensitive. Therefore, he didn't think it was what you should do at any stage. He says that you don't really talk about feelings; you feel as though you have to be the provider and safe haven, and you cannot be seen breaking down when you are supposed to be the one picking up the pieces. I asked if he grieved after the miscarriage at all, and he said he doesn't know, probably not.

His words were, "I don't know...I'm not very in touch with those things. I'm getting a lot less emotional the older I get and brush a lot of them off. After years of loss and hurt, you learn to think that this is just the way things are. It's not a good thing, but I just shut that stuff off." He felt that he didn't have the right to grieve our loss because he wasn't carrying the child.

He says it's mainly just the mother feeling this physically, after creating that bond. Mel feels that yes, as the man, he has something to grieve about, but you can't really talk about it. He was more worried about me than anything else, and he was concentrating on my well-being. He tried his best to put me back together; that's where his focus went.

We have a family friend who is a priest. He married us too. We met up with the priest in Mel's sister's house one day, and he offered his words of sorrow for us. He was most sincere and genuine. He asked me if I was ok and not to worry, that a little baby will come for us, and he can give his word on that. He was one of the first to ask me if I was ok. I was so glad, as I wasn't used to that.

He also approached Mel and said that he was sorry for our loss, a life is a life, no matter how early it was, and things can be cruel. He reassured us that he was praying for us and could see that a child was meant for us. He was the first and only person, who uttered the words, **"Sorry for your loss,"** followed by, **"How are you?"** He spoke to us, and he truly believed and understood the sense of loss that we carried. He has seen it time and time again. We valued that massively, and we still talk about that.

Chapter Sixteen

It was now coming near the end of November 2022. I was still living out the two week wait periods in despair. The two weeks wait (2WW) is one of the most mentally draining things you'll ever experience. It is the period of time between ovulation and the day of your expected period. I was busy checking for mucus, trying to see if my cervix was opening, checking my temperature, logging every twinge, going to the gym, taking the prenatals, and a probiotic, being mindful of food, so on and so forth. This was so draining and exhausting. I was peeing on ovulation sticks and beckoning poor Mel to the room once again. I was very low; I was just existing and functioning, but I was not happy. I was totally drained and fed up. I was losing all hope. I spoke to a friend who told me about a lady called Caroline, who she had heard about, who was meant to be good at reflexology to help you to get pregnant.

    She knew someone who went to this lady, and after her first month of going to her, she got pregnant. I mean, I hadn't even considered this before. I wasn't really into these alternative medicines or airy-fairy things, as I once thought, but I was out of ideas and energy. I decided to give it a whirl. What was there to lose?

    It was a sad, dreary, evening in late November, and I decided to give Caroline a call. She couldn't speak just then, so she said she would call me back, and she did. After just two minutes of general chit chat, I felt as though I liked her. It felt right and not forced. She seemed genuinely interested and knowledgeable. She asked me why I was calling her, and I explained that I had a miscarriage and was feeling incredibly mentally stressed from it. I also mentioned that we were trying for a baby again, but nothing was happening, and that I was at my wits' end (whilst half crying down the phone).

She asked me what day of my cycle I was on, and I told her. She asked me some general health questions and about my mental state, and then she issued the following instructions. She said that she was happy to see me, but asked me to wait and see if I got my next period. She wanted to see me on day 1 of my next cycle, and it didn't matter if it was on a Sunday or when it was, but to let her know straight away so she could arrange to see me that day.

She was so kind and reassuring as she said, "If it has to be late at night or first thing in the morning, I don't care. But I need to see you. If you wake during the night and have gotten your period, send me a message, and as soon as I get it, I'll call you with an arrangement." She explained her usual course of treatment would be for me to visit four times in that month; on days she assigned. She said she'd give me some basic instructions to follow and offered her kindest sympathy to me before we ended the call.

As the days passed by and the due date for my period loomed, the anxiety kicked in again. I wondered if I was pregnant. Should I take a test just to see if anything shows up? Will I stop drinking coffee just in case? Maybe I should ease off in terms of movement. I was checking fluid, analysing myself for twinges, and really trying to be in tune with my body. I was searching for signs and symptoms in my head. In fact, I'm pretty sure I was making up some symptoms to convince myself it was a possibility. The mind plays many a trick when you are anguished. I was almost delusional. I was trying to do meditation and relaxation all while thinking about a million different things in my head, while pretending to myself that I was relaxing. It is just not for me!

And then, there it was...my period again, at the very end of November. Talk about being flattened. I was going to see Caroline that evening, and I had no idea what to expect. I went inside and was greeted by a smiling, reassuring country woman. She was strait-laced and just a regular person. She didn't fit the stereotype that I had in my head. She asked me some questions and then asked me to get up on the bed so she could look at my feet and body. She started reflexology, and I said, "This is where I'll close my eyes now and relax." She said to go ahead and relax. I was lying there, and after about two minutes, she stopped and said, "Ok, I'm sorry now, but you think that you are relaxed there, don't you?"

I opened my eyes and was looking at her, confused. She stood back, looked at me, and said she hasn't seen someone so tense in such a long time, as I lay there with my arms and legs poker-straight, convinced I was relaxed. She was right; I spent all my time telling myself to keep my eyes closed, think of a black space only, and try to relax. Basically, all I could hear and focus on was this voice in my head asking me if I was relaxed yet.

Caroline said that we would just chat as she is working on me, and to be fair, within minutes, I could feel my body relax a little more. She assessed me from head to toe, and we discussed some things such as nutrition, sleep, and relaxation. What really struck me was the fact that stress is such a major factor in reproduction. In a nutshell, she described me as living in fight or flight mode. I am always thinking, "What do I have to do next? Where do I have to go?" There is never a dull moment, there is never time to just do nothing. I was, and still am, always planning and organising something to my detriment. She explained that the release of cortisol into the body (a stress hormone) tells the body that it is not a good time to get pregnant, as the environment in the body is not welcoming or appropriate for a baby. Therefore, nature has a way of knowing when the timing is right or not.

She also enlightened me that it is also thought that your mental health dictates a lot of the body's responses to what we think are natural things, such as pregnancy. If you live in an anxious state, the body can sense that and, again, can prevent pregnancy from happening. I must say this all made sense to me. She explained it better and, in more detail, but I already knew going in there that the only thing getting in the way of a successful pregnancy was my head and my obsession. I just had a feeling. Any overexertion on the body can have the same impact, including rigorous exercise or a diet too low in calories and many other attributes. That is my understanding, anyway.

I was living life in the fast lane, keeping so busy in order to distract myself. Between that and the scheduled intercourse, injections, ovulation tests, pregnancy app obsessions, and early testing before my period, it was relentless. Add to that the mucus checking, the endless online searching for answers, the multiple scans, physical examinations, and blood tests, so on and so forth. It is no wonder my body had a block against pregnancy. Nature is very clever, you know.

So, it is that simple...don't stress! Yeah, sure thing, if only. Caroline introduced me to grounding and deep breathing. The first time I did the breathing with her, I felt my body decompress breath by breath. To my surprise, it was heavy, as in relaxed and not as tense. My arms and body felt heavy, and my shoulders dropped back. She explained the different combinations of oils she'd used, and she sent me home with some of the remaining oil, with instructions for use, self-care, slowing down, and doing the practising breath work.

At each appointment, she gave me oil blends that she makes up specifically, but one ingredient that she spoke about was clary sage. I am no expert on this, but I do know that it is not something to be messed with, without professional guidance. You are not recommended to drink alcohol with it, and it can be used to cause contractions to ensure clearance during a period, and also in early labour. Professionals use the correct levels of it in the right blend.

One of the active ingredients in it increases oxytocin, which in turn, when used correctly and under guidance, can encourage uterine contractions while also reducing any spasms and relaxing other areas of the body, allowing the reproductive system to balance and clear. It also plays a small part in relieving pain. So please DO NOT MESS WITH THAT ONE.

Caroline told me over the phone and in person the first time I met her, that she cannot guarantee that I would get pregnant, but she does an initial assessment with people and will decide from there if she thinks that she can offer genuine help or not. She doesn't continue to see people for the sake of filling up her book with appointments; she truly believes in her work and always strives for her clients' success. I left there feeling like a tonne weight had been lifted, in a comforting, grounding way. I had finally relaxed, and I couldn't wait to get home and tell Mel all about it and go to bed.

Caroline gave me certain dates that I had to go to see her, in line with my cycle. On my second visit, we chatted about the miscarriage in detail, along with general life. It was almost like counselling as well, to be honest. The rest of the visits were much the same. I had become more aware of myself in terms of being able to feel anxiety coming on and being able to go and do some breaths and calm myself back down. I was much more mindful of looking after myself and trying to relax and sleep more. I also tried to limit the use of apps and Google searches; that didn't always go so well but, I did try. I just kept hearing her voice in my head saying, "Fuel the body like a car."

Fuel (healthy nutritional food), oil (healthy fats), and water. She told me that the one thing that anyone can do safely is to get off any fad diets, feed and nourish your soul and body. She describes our bodies like biological machines that run best with fuel, oil, and water. Our bodies are designed to heal and reproduce, and no matter what the issue is, we will always function better when we give our bodies what they need. That includes movement and rest.

I remember one time she was working on my feet, and she said my uterus was good and busy. I thought to myself, how the hell can she tell that? She could identify that I had a history of kidney infections and could describe my personality precisely.

I often questioned what kind of wizardry she was carrying out until I learned to trust the process. She also does Reiki. She said she often does Reiki as she does reflexology. Some of the times I was there she ended the sessions with Reiki and I used to get an intensely relaxed sensation from that.

Caroline told me to contact her the minute I find out that I was pregnant, and she said she had a good feeling about this. I left quietly confident but also reminded myself of the very real possibility that nothing might happen.

The course of treatment then ended after a month. Caroline usually expects to see success within or up to three months after the full course of treatment, but she also said that it is not uncommon to become pregnant within the first cycle after it.

Caroline was the driving force behind this book as she initiated the conversation on authorship. I remember coming out of there thinking, "That one is mad," where the hell would I be going writing a book, and I laughed it off. She had spoken to me about the fact that she sees so much of this happening and deals with a lot of clients with fertility issues, and it is alarming. She referred to it as a silent epidemic.

It was now Christmas, and I should have been blossoming. I should have been 7 months pregnant, round as a ball, and had a valid excuse not to cook or clean up after dinner. What happened was that dinner was arranged for Christmas at my parents' house. I was on ham cooking duty. I got up early Christmas morning to be greeted by my period. Happy Christmas to me, yeahhhhhhh. I was crampy; as a rule, I don't generally take medicine unless I need to. So, I decided to take paracetamol for the cramps so I wouldn't spend the day being reminded about the fact that I wasn't pregnant. But I accidentally took the opioids that I had been prescribed after the shoulder surgery. They were also in a blue and white box, and I just didn't think. I was meant to finish the course, but I only took it for 5 days because I was high as a kite, and I didn't like that.

Mel had gone to visit his sister, and after about an half hour or so, boom...something came over me. I was dizzy, I felt hot, I got sick from the bottom of my soul...I then checked the box and realised...once I puked a few times, I was fine, but I got a fright. I didn't want to call Mel to come home because I was starting to feel ok again. I was a little freaked out, but I also laughed about it. It was a genuine mistake. I was nearly afraid to drink a glass of wine that day.

My sister was going to drop us off at home from my parents' house, there was no panic on us to go home early she had said, as she was in no hurry. On the day, we had dinner, sitting and sipping away, chatting. The craic was just getting going at around 6:30 pm, and my sister said she was going home. We had to go home because we hadn't prepared anything for the dogs and couldn't just decide to stay overnight at my parents' house. I won't lie; we were kind of raging. Not with my sister, but the fact that this meant we had to go home to an empty, sad house, and spend the rest of the day thinking about how things should have been so different. How they should have been so much happier.

We got home after a quiet journey and came inside. We said, "Ok, let's have a few more drinks and try to keep the fun going." We had such a laugh, we made cocktails with random bits in the press and sat drinking shots and playing card games. Suddenly, it was 1 am and we were fairly tipsy. The tone changed, and the floodgates opened once again. The sadness crept back in. We ended the night on a low, talking about how things should be and how excited we would be if things had gone to plan. We also imagined what I might have looked like with a bump, and how I should have been posing proudly in front of the tree for a photograph. We spoke about what we would have done in preparation for the baby if it had come along. The joy of Christmas was certainly swept away in one clean swoop.

These were the strongest, most painful feelings of sadness and loss. It is so hard to describe, it's such a sense of emptiness, defeat, failure, and complete anger at the world. It's so ironic, because yet again it feels like nobody even noticed or thought about it for one second, yet we were totally consumed with it. No one acknowledged that it would be a hard day, no one thought about our baby, but it's all we thought about. That is one of the things along the way that hurt the most.

Everyone just got on with things; life carried on, but just not for our baby, our hopes, and our dreams. We usually put up the Christmas decorations quite early and take them down early, but that year we couldn't wait to get them down and out of sight. We took them down the day after St Stephen's Day and tried to move along as best as we could.

New Year's Eve came along, and we were not bothered about going anywhere; however, Mel's sister kindly invited us to her house, and we did go. Better to be there than at home wallowing in self-pity. We rang in the New Year, but it didn't feel like there was much to celebrate, to be honest. Yet another night where I cried myself to sleep.

After a few days, my period was gone, and the Christmas and New Year's celebrations were well over. All the decorations were put away, and we had a clean slate for the new year. And with this, we had a new wave of energy. I was on the first cycle after starting reflexology. The golden month, as I called it. This could only mean one thing: it was time to check the app, check the mucus, check the temperature, use ovulation tests, update twinges, and all the usual monthly check-ins that had become a part of everyday life. I was much better at catching myself stressing and calming myself. I was walking lots, going to the forest for fresh air, back to the gym, and making sure I rested in the evenings. What I thought was ovulation came and passed. I was keeping an eye on the app for my next due date for my period. I was curious this particular month because I knew one other person who had gotten pregnant on the first cycle after being with Caroline.

Several times, I had little thoughts where it crossed my mind that I could be pregnant as I endured the two week wait once again. I was trying to be good and wait it out, but I couldn't help myself.

The day before my period was due to begin, I decided to do a sneaky test. I couldn't tell Mel because I was even embarrassed at this stage; it was beyond obsession. I felt like he would either judge me, think I was absolutely mental, or scold me because I had promised I wasn't going to do that sort of stuff anymore. I was going to try to relax!

I had ordered a massive pack of ovulation test strips and pregnancy tests in the early stages of all of this, and I had two pregnancy tests left. I peed on the strip and left it down while it soaked in. I got distracted doing something else. I looked back and saw it was negative. But then I looked again and I thought I could see the faintest line. I mean, it was almost like a shadow. I couldn't even be sure if I was seeing something. Well, talk about examining it with my eyes peering open in full-on binocular mode!

My mind went into overdrive. I tried looking under a different light, I rested my eyes and looked again in case I was imagining things. Then, in one of my most obsessive, borderline psychotic episodes yet, I remembered other women in discussion forums, who in desperation, had mentioned that if you are unsure about the test, you can take inverted pictures on your phone. This way, if it is a positive, you will see it, and if it is an evaporation line or a false positive, it won't show up. For anyone as novice as I was, an inverted picture changes the colouring to look like an old photograph, and if you have a decent smart phone, you can do it too. It doesn't have to be a very fancy model. So, I did that, and I was sure I could see something, but again, it was so faint.

    I was so afraid that it was an evaporation line. I must have analysed it for an hour. I hid it then and went up and down so many times to check it. Mel must have thought I had the runs, or more like he didn't even notice. I know you should only take the results of a test within the timeframe recommended on the box, not an hour later, but I just had to check again. It still wasn't very clear, and the chalky stuff on the strip was drying out, and to my horror, it flaked off! I could no longer see anything on the test. My head was wrecked beyond belief. I was nervous, anxious, excited and terrified all in one. I decided to save my last test for the morning, to keep it for my concentrated wee (IYKYK).

Chapter Seventeen

17th of January: We got up as usual, and I still hadn't said anything to Mel. I couldn't wait for him to leave for work so I could continue my sneaky mission. No offence, Mel. He had to leave before 7 am. The minute the car moved away from the door, I ran to the ensuite and peed on that strip. I had been holding it in until he left. I left the strip down and walked around the bedroom frantically. I went back into the ensuite and took a look. There was a faint line on this one. It was faint, but I could certainly say there was something there. My heart skipped a beat...or two—or ten. I was so excited but also petrified at the same time. My tummy took off with nervous but happy butterflies. I couldn't stop looking at it, I couldn't stop checking. I gathered myself, got ready for work, and headed off as happy as could be. I still didn't tell Mel. I was afraid to believe it, so I decided that I would go to work and get a few tests in the pharmacy to confirm it with Mel that evening after work.

I got home and walked through the kitchen at 90 miles per hour and said, "Mel, come with me, we have to pee on a stick, I have a good feeling." He was cooking and looked at me, confused. He said, "What?" I replied, "Just turn off the food and come with me quick." God love him, he had no idea what I was ranting about. I went to the loo and as I was there, I told him, "I have a good feeling about this, and I hope I am right." We sat and waited for the test to be processed. I could see the fear in his eyes. We spoke and reminded ourselves that if it is negative, we will just try to keep going. We turned it over, and there it was, the double line that we had so longed to see. It was positive. We were absolutely thrilled, but I couldn't help but notice Mel wasn't half as reactive as the last time. He was shocked. He was sceptical and mostly afraid that the same thing would happen again. I was weirdly calm, not anxious, but immensely happy. I knew it was very early as I was only due my period that day.

    Mel really tried to speak to me, reminding me that it was very early and to try not to get too used to the idea until it's confirmed. I was so miffed with him that I couldn't understand why he wasn't excited and was almost bringing negativity to the whole thing. Now I get it, I understand his fears. He was terrified that I wouldn't be able for it again, and he was right, because it had been a shit show up until now. We spent the evening chatting, and I was smiling from ear to ear. Mel didn't say too much. And so began my new obsession with Google searches again. I was searching for the probability of having another miscarriage and all sorts of things.

<u>The loss of a little life really proved to be a thief of joy and provider of fear. Would this be a sticky baby or would it end in tears again?</u>

When we had the miscarriage last time, the GP told me to make sure to visit the EPU the second I got a positive test. I told work I wouldn't be in the next day, and Mel also took the day off. I'm glad he did, because it snowed hard that night. We woke up and headed off to the EPU to have the pregnancy confirmed. We went to a different hospital this time (thank God for choice, eh?). We were lucky to make it. The car got stuck in the snow when we were pulling out of a junction on a back road, but we made it. We were optimistic and excited. We sat in the waiting room to be registered, and when the nurse came in, she said we had to have a referral. I called my GP and she sent a referral within minutes. The nurse was lovely and helpful. She had asked why we were there rather than at the GPs to confirm the pregnancy, and I told her about the miscarriage. She couldn't have been more helpful and kind. We didn't really know what to do or what to expect.

We were taken into the room to be assessed. My bloods were taken to check the HCG levels. This would have to be repeated to check for an increase in HCG, which usually doubles every day or so, which would indicate that pregnancy is developing. I had a scan and I recall there was a very small indication of a pregnancy sack. We headed off home happy, as a pregnancy had been detected in theory, and we would receive a call later that day to confirm the blood results.

Talk about time standing still again! I watched the phone so closely. I kept checking the screen, the volume and the coverage to make sure I didn't miss the call. I just HAD TO KNOW.

The phone rang. The HCG level was 32 mIU/mL. Anything above 25 mIU/mL is considered a strong positive pregnancy test. So that was it. I was certainly pregnant again. Wahoooo. I asked them about starting the progesterone that, earlier, the specialist had prescribed, and they said to start it right away. The relief. Now we had to go back for more bloods in two days and repeat the process to ensure that the HCG was doubling. We did that, and it had jumped to 70 mIU/mL. The numbers got bigger and bigger, and then after the fifth time testing, the nurse called me to say that they are very happy to suggest that this pregnancy appears as though it is very safe at this stage, and it is off to a perfect start. They advised that I relax, reduce stress, and take extra care of myself every day.

I had already collected the progesterone from the chemist when I got my injections months earlier, so I had them ready to go. I was excited that night to have an early night and start the progesterone. This was going to help maintain the pregnancy. I opened the packet, and there was a long applicator. Longer than a tampon applicator. I inserted the progesterone and lay still for half an hour to let it dissolve as per instructions. Thankfully, it didn't hurt. It was a mighty excuse for early nights. This had to be done every morning and every night for the first four months. Mel was very good; he brought me tea and toast to keep me going before he went to work, as I had to repeat the process every morning. He is always loving and caring, but even more so now.

This pregnancy brought up a lot of emotions for us both. I really started to think again about the loss we already had. I had said to Mel that we need to start thinking about jazzing up the memory tree at the front and add some flowers to brighten it up. I wanted to plant flowers timed to bloom around the baby's due date in February. We agreed that we would get some and try our hand at being green-fingered. We planned to go in the next three weeks and get some flowers.

I had forgotten that one of my friends had booked in to see a fortune teller/medium and invited me along. I was only four days post-positive test on the day that we headed off. We met up and all travelled in the one car. We agreed that when we came out, we wouldn't ask each other questions until the person who just came out got to take notes, or until they felt like telling some of the stuff that was discussed. I had never heard of this lady before. I had been to see other fortune tellers and mediums a couple of times, as I find it intriguing. I always go to them with scepticism, but usually they say something that grabs my attention.

The appointments were booked by one girl who used her first name, and my name wasn't even given. The two other girls went in first. Finally, it was my turn...

She greeted me at the door and said hello. Then she said, "Oh God, you have such a heart of gold, don't you, you are a very good person." She then beckoned me inside and stood looking at me for a second and said, "Come in and tell me all about the loss...there is a miscarriage here, isn't there?" At that, I started crying (surprise, surprise). All I could think about was how the hell she knew that in the space of a few seconds. She walked me to the couch, and I sat down, taking a tissue from the box.

She started to talk about it some more. She asked me when did it happen and I told her. She said, "Oh God, you were absolutely broken-hearted from this." I agreed (naturally, as anyone would be broken-hearted). She asked me, "Have you given the baby a name?" I was totally stunned and embarrassed because I hadn't even done that.

I explained to her that it happened so early that I didn't know if it was a boy or a girl. She looked at me and she said, "Oh, believe me, in your gut you know." She left me in silence for a moment. She said, "I'm going to count to three, and I want you to say any name that comes into your head."

1...2...3..."Dylan," I said. She smiled at me and said I have a message for you from Dylan. He said, "The reason I couldn't stay is because I knew I had some sort of heart issues, and I was either going to leave the earth very soon after birth or live a very complicated and difficult life, which wouldn't really be like living at all. I really don't like needles, like daddy, so I didn't want to have to go through all that medical stuff."

My sceptical side thought, "Hmmmmm, this seems very generic," until she mentioned the part about daddy not liking needles. As I mentioned earlier in this story, he was, and is, kinda a wimp when it comes to them. It's the one thing he cannot stand and would nearly pass out.

She then told me that Dylan knew about the tree and agreed that we should add flowers around the bottom for some colour. Now, I was thinking there is no way she could know this; I mean, it was the topic of conversation for us just days before this, but I hadn't said it to anyone else, only Mel.

Then she turned her attention to comforting me, explaining that these special babies know that they will only have a very short time. They choose their parent(s) so carefully because they know that the parent(s) will cherish them from the second that they know about them, and that their time is going to be so, so short that they will know what it feels like to be loved to the core, wholly and truly. That the parent or those parents can fill their hearts with all that they need before their soul has to go again.

They know that even when they leave, their parent(s) will continue to love and think about them, and that is why they are happy to leave so soon. They are fulfilled by the love they receive in the short time they are with you, in body.

I got great comfort from that, and I hadn't thought about it that way. I had only thought about it as a negative, as being unfair. I only thought about how I must not be suited to being a parent, or how I'm not meant to be one, or that it was my fault. So, I felt some sense of relief, and it was true; I did love him, and I still do, and always will. It gave purpose to the feelings I still had for this little person, whom I never knew. It was ok to still feel strongly for him; I was meant to!! It felt like I might have done him justice, and that he knew how much I loved him, that he was happy and fulfilled, despite having to go far too soon.

The reading continued and was quite accurate, as she hit the nail on the head with many things, including some messages from my mother-in-law and others that I knew. Most of these messages made sense to me at the time. Some of them didn't until I had conversations with people after, and things were clarified. But the last thing that really got me happened when I was leaving. She stood and gave me a hug as I was leaving, and it went on far too long. I like hugs, but this one was uncomfortable.

However, she was telling me that everything would be ok, I would be ok, and to stop worrying. I said, "Ok, great, thank you," and went to leave. She said, "Oh, Laura, congratulations, by the way." I turned to look at her and had a confused face on me. She said, "How long have you known?" I smiled and said, "Known what?" She pointed to her belly area and said, "About the baby," and she smiled at me. I said, "Shhhhh, nobody knows.

I only found out four days ago." She smiled, winked at me, and replied, "I'm telling you; you have nothing to be worried about with this one. Everything will go smoothly, so don't be stressed out. Relax and go home in the knowledge that this is all going to be ok. You and your baby. And this baby is a very special baby. More than you even know. This baby will play an important role for your father and so many others in the time to come." I then turned and gave her a hug. I now became the weird one, not letting go! I could feel her excitement for me. We had some weird moment, a connection I can't quite describe, but it felt like we clicked or something, I have no idea. I was grinning from ear to ear going out to the car, and I had to remind myself not to say too much to the girls in case I gave away that I was pregnant.

Like, how could she know that? I couldn't believe it. I hesitated to trust her that it might all be okay, considering everything that had happened before. Was she right? What would happen next? Would I get my happy ending, or would it all fall to pieces again? Only time would tell.

We followed through with our garden plans and spent a few quid on flowers, feed, weed-stopping sheets, and whatever else we needed after that to plant flowers under the tree. Off I went and planted lots of snowdrops and some other colourful flowers- I've no idea what they were even called. In my mind, the snowdrops would certainly grow because they are so hardy. They disappeared shortly after being planted. However, they do pop their heads up in the spring, in February, around the time that Dylan would have been due.

A year had passed at this stage, and I thought the tree was dead, but thankfully, there are more and more leaves as time goes by. We plan to make a nice seating area here sometime, and we can picture sitting there on sunny days with a family in the future when the tree is bigger. That was the dream anyway.

Reflection

I have spoken to so many women who have endured some sort of experience in relation to fertility difficulties, baby loss, miscarriage(s), or the struggles with the realisation that the dream of having a family may never come true. I have seen Instagram pages and followed real-life stories of people struggling with infertility and IVF, and all the physical and emotional baggage that comes with that. I have spoken to ladies who are sick or have been sick, resulting in them not being able to conceive or carry a pregnancy. I have talked to ladies who have struggled with eating disorders, and as a result, are now infertile. My point is that this is an issue that is happening all around the world and at a growing rate, which is extremely alarming.

To put it into context, **data from the National Library of Medicine in Britain states that roughly 12.5% of women experience infertility. In Ireland, male and female figures are typically grouped together, making it difficult to find an accurate rate for women alone. However, much of the existing discourse and emerging surveys suggest the true figure likely lies between 10% and 20%.**

Trying to conceive isn't straightforward for some. It can mean grieving the life that you expected and hoped for. It can mean feeling left behind as friends and colleagues seem to have no issues. It means endless disappointments

and setbacks, waiting, and longing for that miracle. It brings uncertainty about the future, and can cause you to lose sight of who you are. It can leave you feeling like a fool for believing that this month might be the month.
It means watching your dreams become a reality for others.

As a society, I feel we, in Ireland, need to learn about this and the impacts that infertility, fertility issues, miscarriage, and baby loss have on the people involved and learn how to better support them. Some people brush over it and move on without fuss or a second thought, and that is also ok, but I guarantee you if you ask them how old their lost child would be, they wouldn't have to think about it for too long before having the answer.

Some people do not want to talk about it because the pain is just too much, or they're afraid of slipping back into that dark headspace. What I will say is that many of the people I have spoken to have said similar things about their experience, and that is why I have written this book. This kind of hurt or loss is something you wouldn't wish on your worst enemy. But remember, this could very well come to your door with your mother, daughter, sister, friend, colleague or relative. I think we need to be more compassionate and accepting that this is a big deal to most who experience it. A very big deal.

It is totally consuming and draining, and whether you think someone is being dramatic or not, the least that you can do is offer a shoulder and some small bit of support without being asked for it. A simple text message could make all the difference because for them, this could be the toughest ordeal of their life. Everyone's personality is different, and everyone copes in different ways, and we need to respect that. The important thing is to show empathy.

A loss is a loss, and it doesn't matter how far along you are. AOK Nutrition touched on this when she released a podcast with her miscarriage story recently and she said something like, "A loss is a loss, I came away with nothing, I never felt the kicks, I didn't have a bump or it wasn't seen, but what I did lose was the love, the excitement, the names, and the plans." Anyone I have spoken to refers to this and says they feel that people don't regard the loss as a loss, especially in the very early stages. But it is. I felt that it was insignificant to others and that I was being over the top about it, and should have just moved on.

When you are in the thick of it, this sometimes isn't possible. A loss also includes those failed attempts at conception through medical intervention. Sometimes, this can be multiple disappointments and can cost thousands of euros to try to follow your dream. I was quite surprised by some of the attitudes that I encountered towards this. From talking to some people, I have found that they don't see this as a big deal. It should be accepted, and you should move on. It's just not that easy.

Maybe when that friend becomes distant or doesn't reply, rather than giving out about them or getting mad at them, maybe think about the heartache that they are going through at that time, and if you have not been through it, then you need to thank your lucky blessings. Stop thinking about yourself and go see them, whether they reply or not. Drop off a hot meal at the door and just leave it there. Alternatively, send flowers, or a card, or a self-care basket. Send a text saying that you are thinking of them and let them know that they are in your mind, should they need or want to talk. That costs nothing these days.

For some people, losses, in whatever form they occur, are repeated over and over again. And let's face it, although often completely unintentional and coming from a good place, family and friends can be pains in the ass. What I mean is when they keep asking, "When will ye have a baby?" or something like, "Ye would want to get on about it now," or when family and friends feel that you are ignoring them, but the reality is that you are so deep within the trenches and cannot think of anything else. Offer a kind gesture; you might feel that it goes unnoticed, but that person in the trenches will always remember that. It might just take them a while to come back to themselves, to be able to face humanity again and to thank you. Imagine the concentration of feelings and emotions from repeated cycles of medication, physical and mental turmoil, procedures, waiting and losing all hope along the way with disappointment after disappointment, time and time again. It is soul-destroying.

    For all these issues mentioned, I think it is key that we are patient. Let people deal with things in their own time. Don't pry it out of them; let them tell you if they want to. Be available and let them know you are there if they need to offload. When they do, just let them talk. Don't offer unsolicited advice; offer them kindness and comfort. That's about all most women need at that time. They need to know that you have their back and are happy to listen to them.

Dear Me

I remember you. The version of you who was consumed—utterly obsessed—with cervical mucus, planning, timing, tracking, Googling, hoping. You didn't just want it to work—you needed it to. Your days were built around cycles and apps. Every symptom was a clue, every sensation a potential sign. You weren't just trying to conceive; you were trying to reclaim control in a situation where control was impossible. And it broke you, quietly, slowly.

You isolated yourself, trying to do everything *perfectly*. You thought if you just got it right, it would happen. But it didn't. And you blamed yourself. You felt like a failure, ashamed that something so 'natural' wasn't happening for you.

You're used to achieving things through determination and through action, and you take pride in the fact that you don't often rely on people. But this? This process was different. You couldn't out-work or out-smart it. And the helplessness ate away at you. Stress took over your body and mind. You couldn't focus on anything else. Your world became small, filled with pressure, anxiety, and the unbearable cycle of hope and disappointment.

You wanted people to ask if you were okay. To follow up. To show more care. But they didn't, not in the way you needed anyway. It wasn't out of badness, but people often don't know what to do or say in these situations. You saw others with support circles, thoughtful gestures—visits, cards, warm check-ins, and you wished you had more of that rather than days and days spent alone in misery and despair, left feeling unseen and unimportant. You had love around you, and you knew that, but the silence still rang loud. So you stopped talking. Because it felt like no one really *wanted* to hear. And if they were uncomfortable with the conversation, somehow *you* felt like you were a burden. That made you feel like you had no valid reason to continue talking about your loss and the situation that you found yourself in. You felt like you didn't have a right or a need to keep talking about it as a result. It was like people might think that you were just being a drama queen if you did. But let me be clear now: **their discomfort was never your shame to carry. You don't have to carry the weight of it all on your own.**

You must be kind to yourself. Allow yourself the grace to recover. You are grieving, not just the loss of a pregnancy, but the loss of dreams, of certainty, of control. And if you feel called to give your baby an identity or a name, go ahead and do it despite what others may think. There is no timeline, no rulebook. It was your child, no matter how early you lost it. It's not silly, it's not dramatic, it's *real*. Treat it like the loss of any other loved one. Give it the recognition and acknowledgement it deserves. You felt so hurt that some people ignored or avoided the conversation or didn't bring it up, like it didn't matter or wasn't important.

It is ok to feel that way; it was true to you at that time. It doesn't make you a bad person to desire more support at a fragile time in your life.

Trying to conceive can be brutal on a relationship. I know, because you turned this into a military operation. Schedules. Plans. Timers. But don't forget to love each other outside of this process. Be tender with one another. This isn't a test of performance. It's a journey of endurance. Be human together, not just partners on a mission.

Men and partners are often left out of these conversations, but they suffer too. Your partner also lost a child. They are trying to support you while likely unsure how to process their own grief. Don't forget to check in with *them*. In general, this isn't a solo experience; it affects you both.

This experience taught you more than you ever wanted to know:
1. **You are stronger than you think.** You've fought battles in your own mind and heart that no one else can see. And you're still standing.
2. **Stress matters.** It can take over everything. So give yourself permission to enjoy things. Laugh. Breathe. Rest. It matters more than you realise.
3. **You deserve to live.** Have the glass of wine. Go to the party. Don't skip out on joy because of 'what-ifs'.
4. **There is no shame here.** This is not your fault. You could not have prevented it.
5. **Let go of the guilt.** You were doing your best in an emotional storm. That's all anyone can ask.
6. **Advocating for yourself was brave.** You may have felt broken, but you still stood your ground. Be proud of that.
7. **Anxiety may linger.** But you've survived 100% of your hardest days so far. You can keep going.
8. **Trust yourself.** You doubted yourself so often, but you kept showing up. That's who you are.
9. **Try everything.** If it brings relief—acupuncture, massage, Reiki, long walks, long naps—even if it gives you a placebo effect, who cares, once it comforts you. You're allowed to feel better.
10. **You are a force.** You lived through this, and then you *wrote a book about it* so that others wouldn't feel alone. That's courage. That's generosity. That's legacy. Allow yourself to be proud of that.

You were trying so hard to make sense of something that refused to follow logic. It was a cruel test, and it shook you to your core. You made it through. You're still here. You're still standing. You are not the same woman anymore—you are wiser, softer in some places, stronger in others. You have grown so much. You might find that you cling to faith, of sorts, (which you never expected to happen). Lean into it; it just might give you hope when you feel like there is no hope.

Know this—**your baby only ever knew love and warmth and what it was like to be wanted so badly**. Not fear, not pain...only love.

And finally—**let the guilt go**. It is not your fault. Nobody prepared you for this. Nobody taught you how to navigate the heartbreak, the silence, the trauma. Those haunting thoughts in your head...it's time to let them go. They don't belong to you anymore. **Those images in your head of the day you lost the baby at home—let them go.** They no longer serve you. You've carried them long enough. They are not the proof of your love, your pain, or your motherhood. You don't need to hold them to prove what you went through. Letting them go doesn't mean forgetting. It means choosing peace.

And so now, I bid this version of me farewell. It's time to close off this journey and look forward to what is coming next. Life is a gift, treasure every moment and every person in it. The new 'me'.

With deep love, You—who knows now, what you didn't know then. Laura x

About the Author

Laura is a woman from Longford, Ireland — an Irish woman, a wife, a mother, and a teacher — who, like so many others, has experienced the deep and often silent grief of miscarriage and the heartbreak of fertility struggles. Through her personal journey, she came to realise just how many people around her had gone through similar experiences, often quietly and without the support they truly needed.

She believes that during one of life's most profoundly difficult and transformative periods, often what people need most is to feel seen, heard, acknowledged and understood. Yet far too many walk this path alone, burdened by the invisible pain of loss, longing, uncertainty, and a lack of acknowledgment.

This book was born from that realisation. A belief that, as a community, we must do better in supporting one another through these quiet struggles. It was not written by an expert or medical/health professional, but by a woman who has lived through fertility struggles and who believes in the healing power of shared stories and compassionate connection. Her hope is that readers find comfort, information, understanding, empathy and above all, the reassurance that they are not alone.

Acknowledgments

I would like to begin by expressing my heartfelt thanks to Caroline Luke and Dr. Mary Helen Hensley. Without your encouragement, insight, and unwavering support, this book would not exist. I could never have imagined writing something so raw and personal, but you both saw the value in my story before I did. Your belief in me, and your quiet but persistent encouragement to simply begin — gave me the courage to tell the truth, even when it hurt.

To Conor and Niall of ShadowScript Wordsmiths — I owe you more than words can say. You were more than editors; you were guides, sounding boards, and a constant source of reassurance. Thank you for your professional brilliance, your personal kindness, and your tireless dedication to this project. I always felt held, heard, and understood. I felt in safe hands.

To Susan, my publisher at BookHub Publishing — thank you for seeing the heart of this story and carrying it into the world with care, integrity, and compassion that it deserves. Your support has meant the world to me.

To my family, friends, and colleagues — thank you for believing in me, especially during the times I couldn't believe in myself. To those who did listen patiently when I needed to vent or cry or ramble — your presence made more of a difference than you'll ever know.

To the courageous participants who allowed me to share your deeply personal stories on my website — thank you for your trust. It takes extraordinary strength to speak your truth, and I hope you know the impact your words will have on others walking similar paths. You are part of this book's heart, part of its purpose.

To the bereavement counsellor I refer to as Lisa — you saved me from myself. I don't know where I would be now without your wisdom, compassion, and quiet strength. You helped me find my way back to myself. Thank you.

To those who followed my journey on social media — your messages, your openness, and your solidarity reminded me time and again why this book matters. You helped me keep going. To everyone who shared their own stories with me — your words gave me strength. Thank you for letting me carry them with me.

As for my wonderful husband, Mel — this is your story too. Thank you for holding me up when I couldn't hold myself. You will always have my heart. Thank you for loving me the way you do.

For our cherished, beautiful, funny, strong-willed, loving little girl, Mila. You gave us the strength to continue. You are more special than you will ever know. We love you to the moon and back, forever and always.

And finally, to anyone who has known the heartbreak of loss, the ache of waiting, or the grief of dreams left unfulfilled — this book is for you. My heart is with you, always.

Dedication

For Dylan Doyle, our tiny star who never touched the ground —
You were never held in our arms, but you will always be held in our hearts.
Your brief presence left a lasting imprint, and your absence shaped this story.

It wasn't all for nothing.

You mattered.

You still do.

For Mila, our precious little girl —
You are the light that followed the storm, the joy we never thought we'd feel again.
You brought colour back into our world, laughter into our days, and healing into our hearts.
You are everything we hoped for and more than we ever imagined or dreamed of.
We are so proud of you.

We love you x

I better not leave out Willo, she was there for most of this experience too and is as loyal as they come.

www.ingramcontent.com/pod-product-compliance
Lightning Source LLC
Chambersburg PA
CBHW020416080526
44584CB00014B/1363